Nurture Your Body, Feed Your Soul

Pg. 61 — negative self- talk
— seeds

Camera man story - pg. 75

Planting seeds — pgs- 60 + 61

Shoes - pg. 46

Nurture Your Body, Feed Your Soul

The Spiritual Path to Your Ideal Weight

Mary Bray, M.A.

Writers Club Press
San Jose New York Lincoln Shanghai

Nurture Your Body, Feed Your Soul
The Spiritual Path to Your Ideal Weight

Writers Club Press
an imprint of iUniverse.com, Inc.

For information address:
iUniverse.com, Inc.
620 North 48th Street, Suite 201
Lincoln, NE 68504-3467
www.iuniverse.com

ISBN: 0-595-13038-0

Printed in the United States of America

This book is dedicated to you and your unending possibilities.

You are what your deep, driving desire is.
As your desire is, so is your will.
As your will is, so is your deed.
As your deed is, so is your destiny.

—Brihadaranyaka *Upanishad IV.4.5*

Contents

Introduction xi

Step 1
Fall in Love With Your Infinite Possibilities 1

Step 2
Fall in Love With Your Body 31

Step 3
You are More Than What You Think 46

Step 4
Fall in Love With Spirit 68

Step 5
Set Yourself Free 86

Step 6
A Fast of Negative Thinking 103

Step 7
Live in Love 110

Introduction

This book is a transformation—your transformation. You have tried to lose weight many times before, and by now it has probably dawned on you that the process of losing weight has nothing to do with a diet. Food is not the only reason you are overweight. You have eaten too much and you have eaten too little. You have eaten powders and pills with a hope that something outside yourself would give you a good feeling in your body. Becoming thinner has occupied your time, your energy, and your negative thinking about yourself. It has become an obsession, an addiction. You try every diet, only to find over and over that none of them works.

I know this horror of confusion, because I was fat! Just name a food and I know how many calories it has. I was obsessed, addicted and miserable. I hated myself. What I didn't know was that I was looking for more than being thin. I was looking for love, self esteem and acceptance. I wanted to be free of the prison I had placed myself in. Spiritually I had lost faith in myself, faith in God and faith in receiving help. I knew I couldn't go on alone. Inside I was crying for help! I had lost my power—or so I thought. Was I fat because I had given up on myself, or had I given up on myself because I was fat? How did I come to use food as a substitute for what I thought I couldn't have, for what I couldn't be?

I believe somewhere hidden in those rolls of fat, we all can reunite with our self trust, our self esteem, our self worth to create a beautiful body that is not just thin, but also radiant from the Inside out. This is a body full of spirit, full of energy, full of light, full of love!

What we eat is just one part of the learning offered in this book. This book is not fanatic. It is flexible. Its subject is neither food nor eating.

It isn't our negative eating habits that have kept us overweight. It is our negative thoughts and feelings, about ourselves and others, that have weighed us down. If we forgive the past and let go of our negative thoughts and resentment, blaming ourselves, blaming others, we will let go of our fat as well. We are going to go on a diet of forgiveness. We are going to fast from negative thought. As we release the burdening weight in our hearts, we begin to develop a lightness of being. We lift our Spirits to our own delight. We transform our bodies as we transform our Spirits.

All the resentment from the past has taken our energy away. We can let go of this resentment and release new energy into the present where we are now. The new energy fills our hearts in the very center of our bodies with love. We receive our own Spiritual healing from the battering we have created for ourselves through punishment and guilt. Released from negativity we will be released from the overeating we have done to cover up our feelings of anger and grief. We say goodbye to self pity and self hate, the helplessness we have felt. We will find out what the hunger is really that keeps us emptying the refrigerator without satisfaction. We will face the fear that has blocked our ability to love ourselves.

We will set ourselves free! This is a transformation spiritually, personally and socially. Once we have found our true self we can give to others who are equally as frustrated. When we give love and care to others it comes back to us, reinforcing our newfound love of self. We break the old limitations of our past, much like breaking bread and eating it. We are not powerless. It is only the past, our past actions, and our past thinking that are powerless!

As we free ourselves from the past, fear no longer stands in our way of the future because our fears are only old memories of failure that are gone. In the power and peace of every present moment we release our perfect potential. Forgiveness releases energy into the Now, and in the Now we reshape our bodies into perfect health. We have been killing ourselves in the past, and now we fall in love with life.

This book is not only a book to transform your body. It is a book to transform your Spirit! Forgiveness gives back the condition of unconditional love. It brings us back to our true nature. We are love since the very day we came into this world. God is love! This is a diet of the Spirit for we are physical and spiritually beautiful when we are full of love.

We restore our self worth in order to create a beautiful body. We go to our hearts to find our meaning, our destiny, our creativity, our vitality. It's a new awakening for us from suffering to planting new seeds of wisdom, holding on to our beauty on the inside and allowing it to radiate throughout our bodies. The weight begins to fall off as we glow at the newfound freedom of accepting ourselves.

We are going on a joy ride!

Step 1

Fall in Love With Your Infinite Possibilities

Think back to the last time you fell in love. The excitement, the antici-pation, the tenderness, the trust and amazement that come so abun-dantly—there's nothing else like it. Despair melts in the warmth of new hope. Distrust and fear gives way to openness as your heart goes out toward the object of your affection. All things are possible. All dreams are within reach. You can do anything!

This state of mind is the beginning of change—and this is the state of being you can enter that will help you reach your ideal weight and your ideal Self. Most of us experience the bliss of love only when we fall in love with another person. But what if I were to tell you that you can fall in love with yourself? You can fall in love with a new you, who looks, feels, and believes in a better future.

By loving yourself, you will discover that you are inherently perfect and unique. By discovering your unique physical, emotional, and spiri-tual components, you can learn to reveal and live your uniqueness rather than struggle against it. We do this by understanding

- physical components (food, movement, attention to our senses)
- mind components (emotions, habits, accepting change)
- spiritual components (rediscovering love and our defining desires)
- understanding how these come together in limitless possibilities

1

Intimacy with the Self brings about true healing. Intimacy with the Self is a path to self love. The path to love clears up the mistake that something "out there" is going to give or take something that is not already yours. When you truly find love, you find yourself. You find acceptance and your dreams and desires. Reaching the body of your heart's desire is not about food. Food choices are important, but that is only one component in the path to ideal weight.

So, I want to ask you a question: Are you ready to let go of being overweight? Are you ready to lose those extra kilos you've been carrying for 10, 20, 30, 40 years? Are you willing to open your heart to a new vision of yourself? Are you willing to go deep inside yourself to discover the dreams you left behind? Are you willing to remember who you always wanted to be—and then reach for that vision of yourself? This means nothing less than falling in love with yourself and all your limitless possibilities.

Are you ready?

Hungry—for Love

Why do we want to reach our ideal weight? What is it we are searching for? "Being attractive" is something many people name as a reason to reduce their weight. What does that mean? We want to be "attractive." What do we want to attract? Who do we want to attract? Who do we hope will see us as being attractive?

What does it mean to you to be attractive? To a stranger? To a spouse/significant other? How does it make you feel? Do you feel proud? Do you feel like you've been accepted by that person? Do you feel that person has seen who you really are?

Culture gives us many messages that being attractive is mostly about being physically beautiful and young. But if that were all there were to being attractive, then why are there so many wonderful relationships going on between people who don't fit that mold? Certainly there's more to attraction than a waist size.

The mysterious part of attraction is what I think of as sparks. There are some people in the world we're just drawn to for no apparent reason. We see them, and we don't know them but we wish we did. We meet someone and after five minutes of talking we feel that we've known them for a lifetime. Out of these meetings may come a deep friendship, maybe a romance, maybe a partnership for life, or maybe two beings who "pass in the night" but who will remember each other for many years after. These sparks are Divine sparks of love, and this attracts in a unique and indescribably way.

People who embody love in their attitudes and actions give off sparks of joy. How do we embody love? Food can't do it. Gifts can't do it. Hunting for a relationship won't do it. When we let go of our fears that stand between us and our Divine self. When we let go of the facades that stand between us and other people. When we embrace the idea that we are lovable, then we can love. When we have the courage to embrace our Selves, without judgement, we can connect with other people in a genuine way that makes Divine sparks fly.

Our overweight condition signifies that we are out of touch with these sparks. We're out of balance in every cell. In order to have a new body, we have to return to those sparks, the unconditional love and wonder we felt as children. These new views will be the seeds of our new solutions. We can change our bodies by what we *think* and what we *feel*.

Feeling loving sparks transforms our relationship with food. When we've learned how to satisfy our hunger pains and we know what the hunger really is, then we begin to use food to satisfy what it was made to satisfy—physical hunger.

"What am I really hungry for?"
"What am I feeling right now?"
"What do I need in this moment?"

We have a passionate appetite for life—we just don't know what we truly need to satisfy our insatiable craving for wholeness. A return to self love and self acceptance enable us to let go of extra weight from our bodies as well as our souls. We literally reduce our excess baggage—our ball and chain of self criticism, all those feelings of being "not good enough."

We're hungry for inner peace and a deeper connections with ourselves and the universe. We're thirsty for joy and serenity. By learning how to nurture ourselves with "food of the spirit" as well as a new way of looking at food for the body, we can embrace a feeling of total well being. How do we do this? By gaining a deeper awareness of how we function at an emotional level as well as structurally at a cellular level, so that mind, body and spirit function in harmony.

You're here because you're a seeker. You are here hoping to find something you don't have. But what are you seeking? A secret to weight loss? Some special knowledge that will help you find that sense of physical balance you've probably been seeking for a long time? Maybe you're here seeking support from the group so you can put into practice what you may already have a hunch is the right way to live so you can reach your ideal weight.

We seek because we have needs. We have desires. I need. I want. I hunger. We have longings in our bodies. We have longings in our minds and souls. We want more…but more of what? We may want more food, but we've learned that doesn't really satisfy the hunger. Have you ever stood in front of the refrigerator with the door open asking, "What do I want?" The refrigerator is full, but you sense that what you want isn't in there. It's not outside you. It's you.

Is it possible we really want more of *ourselves?*

Food is an amazing substance. We can't live without it, and some of us have had experiences that show we don't know how to live *with* it! After a full meal, we can feel wholly satisfied...or depressingly empty. What's going on? Is it the food? Or is it our relationship to food? Is it what the food does to us or is it the intention we bring to the food?

Let's open the field wider, and I'll ask again: what are we all seeking? What do you want that's related to your body besides reaching your ideal weight? What do you want that's related to your mind? Your spirit? What do you want that's related to other people?

What Do You Really Want For You?

When we ask our heart questions there comes a subtle feeling throughout our body of a oneness with yourself. It is more than a feeling. It is a knowing. It is also a learning. I can exist here in my own heart feeling and feel peace. This peace passes all understanding into a knowing. This knowing comes from a source that is now really in the body and not in our mind.

This knowing is embodied is when we notice that every year in every season nature unfolds and reveals itself in harmony with every living animal person and plant. We don't even question that; we just know it. The peaceful feeling is knowing this has always been and always will be. We can trust it. We know this when we are still, and we all know the glimpses of wonder at the miraculous universe. We are filled with a sense of Spirit, something or someone, a source or a force that is orchestrating our world even while we sleep. We trust that, as we trusted the warm arms of those who held us as babies. Is there a guiding force that orchestrates and organizes our destinies? I have come to believe this is so.

When we are in the state of reverence and a respect for the process of seasons, a child's development, or having a beautiful friendship, we feel only love, because that is our awareness of unity and fulfillment. It is only when we ourselves jump out of this awareness and begin to have self doubt that our state of being changes. We become conscious of this higher awareness through practice. Consciously experiencing this sense of heart felt love causes it to expand, for everything we place our attention on expands. A glimpse of wholeness in nature gives us a glimpse of wholeness in ourselves, for we are nature as well.

As we begin to ask questions of our heart, we definitely begin to get answers, as the soothing words say "seek and you shall find, ask and the door will be opened to you. We have ideas of there these answers come from in the form of God or higher understanding or Spirit. Words don't seem to contain the essence of this larger than life source. I call it Soul. I call it that because it feels soft and warm and loving. It feels complete and content. In this Soul feeling I don't have to reach outside myself to find gratification. I don't have to eat something, or make a telephone call or run to the grocery store to feel at peace. It is just there, in my heart. In these moments of the heart felt awakening we can think of love and know we are loved. We know at a thinking level who loves us and who we love. In the peacefulness of that knowledge, you and I are love, and so is everyone else. This is more than positive thinking or negative thinking or thinking one person is better than another. We see that at the level of Divine Self, we are all from the same source.

Your heart, in the center of your body, is the symbol of giving and receiving this knowing. And you, as the observer of your heart, feel the knowledge that is flowing. Only love emits from your heart. We all know what a broken heart is. It is a feeling of a loss of a love. We know as well what it feels like to be light hearted. Lightheartedness is the state of love. Even God is love. Those words for me hold the whole concept of Spirituality. It encompasses the energy of the whole universe, the whole God force is love. In order to fall in love with ourselves we come to this knowing…and feel it.

You know how it feels to look at a tiny baby or a precious child taking its first steps. It is a pure feeling of love and wonder. You are taking your first steps at feeling and remembering you are this precious child, pure love and wonder, a miracle of nature unfolding as a tree of yellow, green and orange. We go outside in wonder at the colors. Now we go inside with wonder at ourselves.

Acknowledging our heart center creates feelings of peace. One of our greatest desires in life is to be at peace with ourselves. This peace is our loving state. We can get to this state every day with practicing stillness, quietness even in small bits and pieces. For example, while cooking we can notice the colors of the fruit, the miracle of the perfect segments of an orange with the skin around it protecting it. If we were to think of our bodies as an orange, the vital organs inside being protected by our outer body, our skin. We would never abuse this orange, but would pick it up gently, peel it carefully, and appreciate it with reverence. So too with the awareness of bread and how it was created from flour and yeast, baked in the oven until it smells and tastes so good. We love that bread, that orange and we are together in love with nature and all that it gives to us. Our presence in the kitchen is a loving state. We are included in this love, not standing outside from it. We don't exclude ourselves and say, I love this orange, I love this bread, but I dislike myself. It just doesn't go together. Can it be that growing into new awareness, this soul self encompasses the feelings of love? Yes, of course—if we allow it.

We become intimate with oranges, breads, flowers, and trees as well. We cherish each one. Have we not protected our hearts?

Our memories show us that love can be lost and found, or rather found and lost. Loss and broken hearts have led us to fearing love itself. We thought rejection comes from love even betrayal so we steer our ships, our bodies in the direction of isolation of the heart. If we isolate ourselves inside our bodies, we won't hurt and feel the pain of disappointment.

Yet it is our feelings when allowed to be felt that give us messages of the direction we are going. When we travel in the direction of our desires, our intentions, we can't help but feel good. And feeling good is our greatest desire of all. Acknowledging our feelings asks us to search for meaning. What am I feeling? What is this feeling trying to show me. An example is the feeling of being disappointed with ourselves. In the past we have turned off the love of our selves for disappointment. From disappointment comes fear of losing ourselves so to speak. Losing our sense of being accepted by ourselves or others. We go back to our hearts and ask the questions, what is the message that my feelings are trying to tell me? I have betrayed myself? Have I rejected myself? Have I made a mistake?

When we close the door to our feelings we close the door to the energy that activates our thoughts and actions. Awareness of our feelings leads to sadness, anger, and joy. Without awareness of our feelings we cannot experience love. Our emotions reflect our desires.

Only an awareness of your feelings can open your heart. As children perhaps we were taught not to cry or not to be angry. It just wasn't accepted. What would the neighbors say if they heard you? Without feeling our feelings we turned away from our inner messages, our inner desires. We became prisoners in our bodies.

The story of Adam and Eve is the classic myth of human beings searching and journeying into conscious awareness. The Garden of Eden symbolizes the unconscious bliss, the *geborgenheit* of the child, a feeling of essential comfort. The fruit of the tree of knowledge is the symbol of our separate selves. Adam and Eve ate from the forbidden fruit. They formed another identity different from God. As they realized their separateness they felt ashamed of their bodies. By eating the fruit or entering into participation in life as humans they left the state of divinity or bliss as a child. We know when we are tempted to eat something forbidden we are already making plans to eat it the moment that person is gone. The meaning of Adam and Eve, I think, is you don't have to go outside yourselves to attain true knowledge. You don't need anything more than you already are. You are not separate from divinity.

If we have taken forbidden fruit, so to speak, it is a natural function of the mind to resolve the existence of opposites, good and evil, pleasure and pain. We grow out of the innocent unconscious total lovingness of a child into self awareness. We leave the blissful garden of childhood so we can return to our connectedness to the spiritual source with a newfound awareness. As children we made mistakes and were punished. We learned what was accepted and what wasn't. We wanted so much to be good because that meant mother and father loved and accepted us. We wanted more than anything in the world to have their approval. We were their identity. We were how they wanted us to be. Later as we formed our own identity our feelings showed us we were not like our parents, often not like them at all. We didn't dare tell them for fear of disapproval. As they sometimes disapproved of us we felt their love taken away. We thought we were bad. We even may have lost ourselves, our identity and our acknowledging our true source. We were afraid to be ourselves.

The bliss of childhood showed our connectedness to the spiritual source. We were one with our surroundings, experiencing each new moment. All was one. We also learned life is painful. When father or mother leaves we felt uneasy and anxious. Our learning good behavior and bad behavior caused us to believe we were not good enough just as we were. We became broken off from our previous wholeness and became insecure.

In the rest of our lives we search for our lost wholeness, to heal the wounds of separation. Separation and its loss of security cause fear. Fear is the opposite of love. When we are acting out of fear, we are not in love with ourselves. We are trying desperately to get back to wholeness including approval of others. We feel less than good and we want to be more than ourselves. We think we are bad in the eyes of others, and we feel ashamed in our bodies. Our hearts hurt. I think our hearts are starved of love when we are fearful. We start to run around in circles trying to prove ourselves good. The loss of our own self love, respect and reverence causes excruciating pain, inner pain. We are out of control, trying to control others. We have lost temporarily our Spirit as guilt and fear pierce our serenity. We have forgotten who we are. The innocent child of love struggling with love and fear, guilt and acceptance becomes an adult, writhing in the struggle like a snowball that is gathering more and more momentum, getting heavier and heavier.

Just as Adam an Eve found themselves in this dilemma, this is what happens to all of us. What can we do when we feel like we are going crazy, blocked and immobile both physically and emotionally? We can go back to our heart, to our stillness inside, to our knowing, to our reverence with nature, to our oneness with all living things, to asking questions to listening to our emotions wondering what they mean asking questions to the great unknown, to our spirit inside, What does this mean? Where have I gotten off track? How can I get back on to create for myself all that I desire, all that I love about myself?

Trust Your Inner Vision

I truly believe that we all have the power to change our lives, because as human beings, we can make choices. We can let that power sit unused, or we can use our choices to change a negative situation into a reality that reflects our inner desires. This is how we become fulfilled. This is how we reach out for pleasure and satisfaction in life.

The reality and power of thoughts and choices can create change in your life, if you're willing to listen and trust your inner vision. You can do anything you desire with a scale, with kilos, or calories if you're willing to discover the real you and accept all the parts of yourself you may be rejected or betrayed.

This discovery comes from your inner being. As new thoughts, intuitions, and choices come, you will let go of old habits and beliefs that make you miserable. As you make positive choices that open your heart, you feel a new self acceptance. Believe in your vision of yourself as a person at her ideal weight, and you will reach your ideal weight.

I want to tell you a story about myself. This is a story about being overweight. This is also a story about love, acceptance and change.

For years, my extra weight ran my life. I didn't make choices—my fat made choices for me. From the clothes I could wear, the places I felt comfortable going, the people I felt uncomfortable being around…I tried every diet, pill, and program that came along. I used laxatives and diuretics. I went up and down the scale—a typical fanatic yo-yo dieter.

During one point when I was thin, I fell in love. I felt so great about myself, cared for and accepted just as I was. We got married, and I thought all my troubles were over. With love in hand, I thought "This is what I've always wanted. I don't need anything but him and the attention he gives me. Now I have all the love I've always needed. I'll never overeat again to fill that hole. This is the end of the diet road and the doorway to bliss!" I felt loved and accepted just as I was.

Then I started cooking for my new husband, and you can guess what happened. All the weight that new love had taken off promptly came right back on. I couldn't imagine how anyone could want me. It's no surprise that we eventually got divorced. I still had my sense of self worth tied up completely with the number on the scale or what clothes I could fit into. The size of my body was my only measurement for feeling worthy of love.

Then one day, in the early 1980s, I was at the beach with a friend. I was living in Houston, Texas, at the time and since the ocean was nearby, Nancy and I went there often to soak up the sun and find some relief from our hectic lives. I always complained about how fat I felt in my bathing suit. At about 85 kilos, I bulged in all the wrong places. I must have complained every week for months until, finally, Nancy said,

"How much longer do you need to carry that extra weight around? You keep complaining, but you don't take responsibility for losing the extra weight. Why?"

It was a question I had asked myself before but had never really given enough thought to. It's so much easier to keep complaining. As I thought about it, though, I realized that food had a huge power over me. It was a terrible feeling. I was out of control. For some reason, her question hit me hard. For the first time, I really saw the truth: I was doing this to myself. I was the one who was making me miserable.

I was working at a chronic pain clinic at the time, teaching patients to use biofeedback for relaxation and—believe it or not—weight reduction. Here I was telling other people how they'd feel so much better and be so much healthier if they would just lose some weight. I was giving all that advice, and I was overweight! They looked at me, and I know they were asking themselves, "If she thinks this advice is going to work for me, why hasn't it worked for her?"

The next day, I went to Dr. David Axelrad, the director of the chronic pain program. David was my friend as well as my boss, but I still had butterflies in my stomach when I told him, "David, my eating is out of control, and I don't know what to do. Help me!"

He said, "Sure. Mary, are you ready to lose the extra weight?"

I took a deep breath and nodded. "Yes, I'm ready."

Then he asked, "How do you know you're ready?"

"Because I'm miserable," I said. "I want this overweight story finished in my life!"

He told me he could help. He looked so calm and seemed so sure that I could do it. I certainly didn't feel that way myself, but in that moment I took a leap of faith. I decided to trust that he could really help me. I decided to trust that after 30 years of diets and plans that didn't work, this time and this way would work—if I let it.

I felt like a hundred kilos of armor dropped off right there. I felt vulnerable and scared, but I also felt so much lighter inside. I had just told my boss that I was out of control, and he was still looking at me with the respect and caring he always had. He still accepted me—even after I admitted I was less than I wanted to be. We went into his office, I sat down, and he asked, "Can you form an image of yourself at the weight you've always wanted to be?"

I closed my eyes and saw myself wearing white shorts and a white T-shirt. I was on a warm, sunny beach with seagulls wheeling high overhead. My hair was long, and the Mary of my dreams was running toward me. I let the image continue, and soon tears started rolling down my cheeks. After 30 years of denying how wonderful I could really make myself be and feel, I was finally allowing myself to see my possibility. For years, I had believed that I could only be overweight.

I wanted so much to let all the feelings of this new vision become real in my life!

Then David said, "Now see yourself in the past with too much weight, and notice how this seemed to be beyond your control." I saw myself with tight clothes, remembered the broken zippers and buttons popping because my body was bursting at the seams. I felt the total frustration that came with too many years of overeating. At that time, I didn't understand all the reasons for letting myself become overweight and stay overweight, but I trusted my feelings. I knew I wanted the joy I felt in my vision of being thin. I also knew I didn't want the frustration of being overweight.

I surrendered myself to the new learning with openness and blind trust. I was ready.

How Did We Become Overweight?

Before we can move forward, however, we have to understand what has been keeping us back all those years. Where do our eating habits come from?

Our brains store all of our experiences and emotions and play them back to us. How do you eat? What do you eat? Why do you eat what you eat? What do you believe about your own happiness? What do you believe is possible in your family? In your work? In your future? All these questions are automatically answered by your internal memory when certain external trigger them.

These memories are accumulations of experiences from childhood. How we acted with our families, with our friends, in school, and onward—all are deeply embedded. They form the basis for all our behavior today. These memories often play in your head by themselves. Have you ever come home after a busy day and found yourself staring into the refrigerator? Maybe you're hungry, maybe you're not, but you're there…staring at the food. The memory is on automatic play, turning on a habit that keeps the extra weight on and keeps you feeling out of control.

From our earliest years, we form thoughts about food and eating. We do this in order to meet our basic needs for survival. As infants, we communicated our need for food by crying. When we cried we usually also received love and warmth along with food. Early in life we learn that pleasing the person who feeds us (usually mother) gets us approval. We feel good, loved, and nurtured.

This is when the association between food and comfort begins for most people. As a child, did you ever refuse to finish everything on your plate? Do you remember sitting in front of those few bites you just didn't want to finish? Whether it meant not playing with our friends or simply being called a bad boy or girl, we learned to associate bad feelings with not cleaning our plates. As children, we realized the importance of receiving love and positive reinforcement, so we usually ate to please, regardless of whether we were hungry or liked the food.

It doesn't help to blame our parents, because they taught us based on what was in their memories. Well-meaning parents think they are inspiring their child to be healthy. But, as a result, we were often persuaded to eat more than we physically needed in order to earn the reward at the end of the meal...dessert. This all happened while our basic thought and behavior patterns were developing. It is also when our eating patterns and behaviors were developed.

As we became adults, we could decide what to eat or not eat, but we weren't really making choices—we were living out our childhood patterns and memories. But we are so much more than our accumulated habits. As adults, we have the opportunity to learn that to be whole human beings, paying attention to the interconnections of our body, mind, and spirit. We can celebrate the different aspects of our being working together, just as we celebrate the interconnectedness of our own lives with the lives of others. We can think about nutrition instead of counting calories. We can focus on life instead of on controlling food. We can listen to our own hearts instead of only listening to what others tell us.

So how do we change so many years of patterns of thought and eating? Our habits run so deep that sometimes it seems like we were born with those habits in the same way we were born with a mouth. That may feel true right at this instant, but remember—we were also born with a heart, mind and soul. We have a connection to a higher wisdom that guides our destiny. Our hearts and minds hold visions of this higher wisdom that I believe are true reflections of who we are and who we want to become. You'll find out more and more through this book that your ideal weight has less to do with food than it does with this higher wisdom. Those visions are truer than anything we will find in the refrigerator or on a dessert cart.

When my three boys were growing up, it seemed like I lived my entire life in the kitchen. I always had certain foods in the house so I could make their favorite sandwich or snack. But even after they were gone from home, I would still find those foods in my cupboards, even though I didn't eat them. How did they get there? I was shopping from those years of habit instead of by what I needed that day to create my new self.

Eating that leads away from ideal weight is sometimes a matter of old habits. Sometimes we eat to cover up emotions that we don't want to face. I remember one time when I was dieting (before I knew better), eating such small amounts that I was literally starving. I had this overwhelming desire to eat and eat. What did I want? Potato chips with sour cream dip, alternated with chocolate chip cookies, back and forth until all of it was gone. I felt so guilty afterward that the next time I had such a craving, I decided I would sit through it and not eat.

Well it happened one day, this strong urge to eat uncontrollably, and I went to the couch to sit it out. I started to get anxious and the craving just got worse. The longer I sat there the stronger it grew. I sat, I took deep breaths, and my anxiety grew even deeper. I had an overwhelming impulse to eat potato chips and cookies. The craving consumed my whole body. I finally burst into tears and cried and cried for I don't know how long. Sometime later I realized I was just staring out the window. The trees were starting to turn yellow. I was in another land conscious wise. The craving was over. I haven't craved chocolate cookies since.

Sometimes we have a craving that is really good for our body. I've noticed that I crave citrus fruits when I have a cold. My body needs the extra Vitamin C for healing.

But other cravings can be a desire for food that drains our bodies of energy. Many of us drink an excess of coffee or cola beverages, even though we know it's not healthy. The answers lie in the question. Why are we craving for these things? What are we really yearning for?

Life *is* yearning. Without desire and yearning, we wouldn't even get out of bed in the morning. We yearn for meaning, love, and the fulfillment of our dreams. We yearn to be more than what we are. Some yearnings are healthy and take us in the direction of our dreams. Other yearnings can take us down a path of darkness.

The natural yearning for inner strength may become a compulsion for power over others. The natural yearning for love can act out as a hopeless attempt to gain approval from others. We have the yearning for self fulfillment, and that can be turned into an obsession with accumulating money and prestige.

Another craving can be the desire to relive memories from childhood, such as the smell of mother's kitchen. I had a client who craved spaghetti when she went to Paris. When I asked her why, she said she didn't know. After investigating further, she remembered that when she went to Paris with her parents, they ate "weird French food," but they said she could eat all the spaghetti she wanted. She was so relieved that she didn't have to eat food she didn't like that her biggest memory of Paris was eating spaghetti.

On a symbolic level spaghetti was the memory of the whole family together on a vacation. She was reliving the memories of warmth and togetherness...a craving we all have. I have a friend Steve from America who asks me to bring him Oreo cookies every time I go to America. Other American friends can't understand why there is no peanut butter in Switzerland. Food can bring up pleasant memories of mother and father giving us all their attention. When my mother made pancakes it was a special occasion, because it took extra time, and she was doing that just for me. Craving pancakes today symbolically means I crave the care and attention I experienced yesterday.

This disconnected relationship between our habits and feelings can be healed. Instead of feeding our emotional and spiritual cravings with food, we can choose a different path. We can learn to feed our body with food and our soul with love. As we begin to let go of the old chatter in our minds, the chatter of memories and old habits, the chatter of anxiety and perfectionism and self doubt, we begin to hear the inner vision that shines from our heart. We can think of ourselves as a vase full of fresh water and beautiful flowers. The flowers are fiery red, orange, yellow, pure white—a vision of energy and light. After a few days, the flowers may begin to wilt. You look at the water and see that it's turned cloudy. Leaves have fallen from the stems and started to rot in the water. The water, in fact, begins to stink. You think you should change it, but you have too much to do. To really fix it, you'd have to take the flowers out, completely clean out the vase, put in new water, and rearrange the flowers. "I'll do that tomorrow. For the moment, I'll just add a little fresh water." So you add a little water to the vase, the nothing really changes. The water still stinks. After a few more days of this, the flowers have really wilted, and the whole vase stinks. The only way to fix it is to start fresh. So you take the flowers out, clean the vase, put in fresh water, and start over with new flowers. Maybe some of the old flowers are really still blooming, and in the fresh water they become alive again.

That water is like our old habits and old thinking. It makes the rest of our lives stink until we decide to clean it out and start fresh. Before you can start anew, however, you have to know what it is you want to bloom.

What do you really want? Your heart is open now, and you are starting new and fresh. That in itself can give a sense of relief. You are becoming aware of how your body is connected to your mind. You can feel the spirit of movement, a higher awareness of yourself than you had before—a heartfelt awareness. You could call it your higher self, or spirit, or nature, or God—whatever you like.

Just as our thoughts are a window to our mind, we can see through the windows into our imagination, the workshop. And it is the desire to act on our thoughts that creates the motion and the movement toward our intentions and dreams. Taking action toward your intentions shows you that you have all the resources inside yourself to feel joyful and peaceful, living at your ideal weight.

Envision Your Ideal Self

Consciousness creates reality...expectation decisively influences outcome.

—Dr. Deepak Chopra

Several years ago, I was working at a Houston hospital, using biofeedback techniques to teach deep relaxation, stress management and weight reduction to patients with chronic pain. Because extra weight puts strain on the body, reducing weight was an important part of helping patients manage their chronic pain.

I was guiding a client into a deep relaxation using visual imagery. Hanging on the wall in the room was a calendar with scenes of Switzerland. I had been there once, and that month's picture of the red cable car climbing toward a summit in the Alps reminded me of how wonderful I felt while I was there. I looked at it from time to time, letting the picture fill me with delight and good feelings.

As I led my client into imagining a pleasant, comfortable and relaxing place where he had been before, I found myself gazing at the beauty of the red cable car against the snowy background. All of a sudden, while my client was visualizing his scene, I also found myself in a deep state of relaxation. I saw a picture of myself in Switzerland walking in the mountains. Clients were walking with me, recovering from their pain in the beauty of nature, breathing the fresh mountain air, and getting well. As I let the thoughts flow through my mind, I began to wonder if this could really be a possibility. My feelings and desire created the thought that this scene could be real.

In the following weeks, my mind went back to this image again and again. My thoughts were growing, and I was getting more and more excited. At the same time, I was afraid. I went to sleep thinking about it and many times woke up with this image in my mind. I began to talk about it with friends, and many of them encouraged me to consider following it through.

The next time I went to Switzerland, I began trying to meet people who would help me with my dream. After a good bit of planning, I decided to take the risk and move to Switzerland. I had almost no money, so I got a job in a souvenir shop selling and engraving Swiss Army knives. After a short time I started teaching English, but I still had my eye on my dream. I took every opportunity I could think of to help me toward my vision.

Three years later, my first two clients arrived in Switzerland from the United States. During their program, we walked in the mountains, breathing the fresh air, while they recovered from their difficulties.

I share this story to show you how dreams and intentions can become realities. The same sequence that got me to my dream of ideal weight also got me to Switzerland, walking with clients in the Alps. A similar sequence of events can be followed to make nearly any intention a reality, whether it's finding a new job, going back to school, or reaching your desired weight.

Desire is a thought with an emotional charge. Desire creates movement towards unleashing a possibility. It opens a new door and literally gives thought a heartbeat. It stimulates a thrust into a new realm and gives pleasure to the beholder. Desire creates a thirst for knowledge that builds momentum in the direction of your intention. A mild interest is usually not enough to carry an idea forward. But desire, like an unquenched thirst, can carry a thought to the well where we find completion and satisfaction.

Our thoughts give us an indication and a glimpse—even if it is ever so faint, at first—of possibilities that, before a certain thought, had never occurred to us before. I want to take you on a journey where you will find the source of your desire to reach your ideal weight.

Ritual: Envision a New You

Sit back in a comfortable place where you won't be disturbed. Then, find an object that is pleasant to look at. This object is familiar to you, perhaps a plant or a picture on the wall. You look at it gently, focusing on it until your eyes begin to blink and start to feel heavy. This is a normal process of relaxation. The more you do this, the more comfortable it becomes, the more you relax, the more you will integrate this learning. This relaxation becomes a time in every day when you are taking time out just for yourself. This essential time creates a step by step process of integration, allowing you to let go of the old patterns of thinking that clutter your mind and take energy from you.

You are more relaxed now and your breathing is comfortable. Your stomach and chest are rising and falling with every breath. The more you practice the skill of relaxation, the better you feel and the more you benefit...everything you are thinking is more clear...you are filled with a free sense of accepting yourself in the moment.

Now imagine you are walking into a movie theater. In front of you is a large white movie screen. It is blank, without a picture. You decide to sit in the front row and wait for the film to begin. That's it...but now a part of you wants to go into the balcony, and so that part of you goes up into the balcony, leaving the other part of you in the front row. See this now in your imagination...walking up the carpeted stairs into the cozy darkness of the balcony.

Now you have the view from the balcony...and at the same time you can see yourself also sitting in the front row. And it's just so relaxing to do this in your own way. The film is about to begin. You settle back comfortably in your balcony seat, watching the film as it starts and also watching yourself in the front row.

The film is about you. You see yourself as a child, four or five years old. You see this child with your family—playing with friends, going to school, growing up, remembering situations and events from special days for the family. You see that sometimes the child is happy and play-ing, and sometimes the child is sad or confused. Allow a few of these situations to come into your mind. Let them play on the movie screen and watch them from your safe balcony seat.

The years pass slowly to the child…school, holidays, brother and sisters sitting around the table talking, fighting, learning, having fun, not having fun. The child—who is you—is growing through the years, sometimes with love and understanding, and sometimes without those precious feelings. You see from the balcony this beautiful child, who is you. And the child grows up in one way or another until today.

The film stops for a moment, and then you see that the film is being rewound. All the scenes go backward into the past, back through the years, back to the beginning again.

Now you come down from the balcony and sit in the front row of the theater. You are going to play the film again. This time you see yourself very closely. This time, you especially notice the wonderful qualities of the child on the screen. Even in the moments that weren't so fun, you have compassion for that wonderful child. And now you have an inter-esting thought…you wonder if it's possible to step inside the screen, to visit your childhood again. Well, why not try it?

You stand up, walk up the stairs onto the stage, and put one foot into the screen…and now the other foot into the screen…it worked! You are back in your childhood. The child in the scene looks at you with sur-prise and delight. The child is so happy to see you. You give each other a hug and a kiss. You take the small hand of the child—who is really you—and you tell her you are here now, and she is safe. Tell her you love her. You realize this child needs you, and you need the child, too. Perhaps you say something like,

I'm here now to comfort you, and I want you to be with me always.

Take the Child's hand and feel it in your hand, bonding in love and acceptance. The child looks into your eyes and feels comforted. Now the movie continues through the years, with you and the child growing up together until this present moment. You can see that this beautiful child is the parts of yourself that you have hidden—the parts that you thought before weren't good enough—the dreams you left behind—the ideal Self who got buried as you grew up.

You know this is a perfectly innocent child, and this part of yourself will help you to find self acceptance. The movie comes to the present moment, and once again you rewind it. This time, you and the Child stay in the film, playing it backward until the beginning…your new beginning, whole and integrated inside yourself.

Now you are ready to imagine a new future. Notice the voices inside that are telling you what is not possible. Set those voices aside. Those voices are silent for the moment, and now anything is possible. Hand in hand with your perfectly integrated loving self, you can gather the courage to look into the future…the future that you are creating.

The movie causes us to remember that sometimes we left our dreams and visions behind. Sometimes we were told that our dreams simply weren't possible. Over the years we came to believe it was too late, or we didn't have what it takes to make them come true. In my seminars many people tell me they forgot to even think about what they wanted…they simply didn't have time…for themselves, that is.

Inside yourself there is a voice or an intuition of what you want for yourself. If you were to imagine that you are free to let your intuition lead you, that small inner voice or insight that gives you a feeling of satisfaction in your heart, what do you really want?

What would you do that would make you really happy? Would you reduce your weight? Would you be able to fit into your favorite skirt, tuck in the blouse? Would you be more creative? Would you learn to sing or paint? Would you fly an airplane? Would you lay on a beach and sleep for three days? Would you fire your boss? What can you imagine yourself doing that would bring you happiness?

Think about these things, and tell yourself:

> *In this moment, I love myself for the possibilities I have inside.*

Just the idea of asking your self "What do I really want?" causes a search through all of your senses. As you keep asking, you get more and more answers. You have to dare to be honest with yourself. When an answer comes, allow it to stay in your consciousness. Write it down. Tape it to your bathroom mirror or the refrigerator, where you'll see it every day.

Like all other seeds, you are going to nurture and nourish these thoughts of your possibilities just like you would if were starting to grow a new little tree. You certainly wouldn't forget about this little seedling would you?

One time in my groups there was a woman named Hedy. She wanted to reduce her weight, but in her depression couldn't find the motivation to act on her desire. I asked her, "What would motivate you?" She said her husband had died a few months before, and she wasn't motivated to do anything. She was grieving, overwhelmed in her sadness. I asked her if she and her husband had something they always wanted to do but didn't in the time they had together. She thought for a moment, and said, "Yes, we always wanted to go to New Zealand."

I said, "Did you have a special Travel Bureau that you used?"

"Yes," Hedy answered.

"I wonder if your travel bureau could suggest a trip to New Zealand for you?" I replied.

She looked shocked at the suggestion. "Oh, I would never go alone! Impossible...Unmoglich!"

"Hedy," I said, "will you do something for me? Telephone your travel bureau next week before you come back here."

She hesitated, but she didn't refuse. The rest of the group also had various tasks they had to pursue toward their long forgotten dreams.

The next week—I'll never forget it—Hedy walked in my course room with a lighter step. She came up to me and said, "I lost one and a half kilos."

I was amazed at her transformation. "How did you do that?"

She said, with a precious smile on her face, "I have registered to go to New Zealand…and I will not go in these 'fat clothes'!"

Six months later and 13 kilos lighter, Hedy was on her way to New Zealand. Out of the darkness of her grief, she found the light that was still waiting for her to live in. She had allowed herself to enjoy those aspects of life that she thought were gone forever.

What do you really want? In the next days and weeks allow your dreams
and your desires to live! Pay attention to them—whatever they are, even the ones that seem "impossible."

The Path of Pleasure

What do all the things you want have in common? How do these things we want make us feel? Do they give us pain or pleasure?

Pleasure, of course. If we think about it in this light, most of our daily life is filled with activities that in one way or another are about seeking pleasure. We want to feel good, and that means feeling good about ourselves. We want to be able to like ourselves, the way we look, the way we act, the way others regard us. We want to feel comfort. We want to feel secure. We also want to be able to help others feel secure. We want to be able to give and receive the most intimate, trusting feelings and live a life that reflects those feelings. We want to be loved.

When we're living and acting out of these pleasurable feelings, we can feel satisfied and become whole. We begin to realize our potential in ways that we never imagined before. We begin to tap into the field of infinite possibilities, where barriers come down and we begin to become the person we have always wanted to be. We find our Perfect Weight, better health, more loving relationships, more creativity…so much is waiting for us. It is there that we can feel and act *fully* human, fully giving, fully loving and being loved.

In much of our world today, however, seeking pleasure is usually seen as a self-centered activity that is at the expense of other people, and keeps us psychologically and emotionally in an immature state. Indeed, if we seek pleasure *only* for the purpose of avoiding pain, then pleasure can become a substance of addiction. If we expect that buying something new is going to solve our relationship problems, we could be unaware of what we really want. If we think that a few cookies will make us feel better, it could be a childhood memory.

So we are going to understand that seeking pleasure is the beginning of a path that brings us into greater connection with ourselves, with other people, and with the Divine inside us. It's a first step toward opening our hearts to possibilities that we can't reach any other way. We can use it as a tool for motivation and it can help us face—not avoid—the difficulties that everyone faces from time to time.

Because life isn't always pleasurable. We all know that. Do we all like ourselves 100% of the time? Do we always do what's best for ourselves and others? Are our relationships always loving? Do we always follow through on our loving commitments to ourselves? Life isn't always so simple. Stress bears down from so many different directions. We may lose a job. We may have to move. Someone we love leaves or is taken from us. We do our best, but we feel misunderstood, even guilty or not good enough. We do our best, but sometimes we feel we haven't done enough.

The disappointment, that feeling in our gut that says things have gone badly, is a horrible feeling. And that can trigger, for many of us, a trigger to compensate that feeling with something that is pleasurable.

When we feel bad inside, it has been a typical response to look outside of ourselves for the answer. For many of us, that compensating pleasure has been food, but it's not what we needed.

The food may make us feel better in the short-term, but as weight is gained and the clothes get tighter, it only adds to our pain instead of supporting our search for pleasure. What's the answer? A diet? You just have to look at all the diets that are available to know that they're not working. Typical diets create a sense of deprivation that feeds pain, not pleasure. Your ideal weight can integrate with your daily life in a way that you can maintain forever. Like the short-term pleasure you get from eating that chocolate in a stressful moment, a diet is a short-term solution that rarely lasts. The weight comes back, and you face the same dilemma as always. This is the yo-yo diet syndrome, and if you've experienced the yo-yo, you're definitely not alone.

So how can you change this cycle? Essentially, this book helps you to deconstruct the old habits and ways of thinking that kept you trapped and help you find the wholeness, acceptance within yourself, and a practical structure for living that supports your ideal weight. Instead of seeking pleasure in food, you can balance that with seeking your heart's desire in all of life.

This isn't simple compensation, trading one sensory pleasure for another. The pleasures you may find in this week are in the realms of body, mind and spirit. To discover them, you'll be asked to explore your own desires and intentions in ways that expand how you view yourself and the world. See your as a seeker of love, a person capable of infinite creativity, fully loving and lovable.

Choose Life in the Direction of Your Dreams

If you knew that it was not possible to fail, would you make the decision now to follow your dreams? Making the decision will change your thoughts into actions. We will explore more about this. Many of the problems in our lives are not the result of wrong choices; they are the result of not making a choice in the first place.

If we decide firmly and resolutely, then we can get what we want. If we flounder in indecision and procrastinate, we lose that ability. In order to create change in our lives, we must be willing to take a definite step in a specific direction. We must decide to risk where we are now for what may be a brighter future. That risk can be scary! The distinct differences between our old way of thinking and our new success can make us feel disoriented and confused. This is normal. It's part of change, and it will fade as you discover the fullness of your being.

Let me tell you about a decision I had to make that wasn't so easy, and I know that you can think of similar situations in your own life. When I decided to come to Switzerland, it meant that I was leaving the safety of the country and language I grew up with. It meant my family and friends would be far away. By going to Switzerland, I was also not choosing to go to California, England, or anywhere else in the world.

We can't be everywhere. We have to make a choice. And to make sure we're making the right choice, we have to be absolutely clear about what is important to us right now. Sometimes, instead of making a decision in a positive direction, we let pain decide what we don't want. "I don't want to feel the pain of change, so I'll stay the way I've always been." "If I ask for help I might feel foolish." But how painful is it to look at yourself every day and wonder why you can't be the person you've always dreamed about? Is your doubt blocking you?

By nature, we do everything we can to avoid pain—both physical and emotional. Have you felt enough pain about your weight? Are you ready to make the decision to change? That means you must rule out all possibilities of remaining overweight. Say out loud, "I will no longer allow myself to be overweight." Remember, we get what we settle for.

As you read this book, listen to what your inner voice tells you. This voice may be faint and hard to hear at first. The more you trust yourself and listen to yourself, the louder and stronger that voice will become. This is the voice of your true desire.

Every decision takes courage, because we face the unknown, we fear the possibility that we might give up on ourselves, we fear feeling like a failure, and sometimes we even fear success. If for any reason you decide that this is not the right time for you to reduce your weight, simply set this book aside and come back to it when you're ready. It is not a failure to respect your own process.

You will be able to read this book in a short time, but this is only the first step. The next step is living the wisdom you find in yourself. It's important that you give yourself time to live with the new learning before challenging yourself with more new ideas. Allow the new knowledge to sink from your brain into your heart, your stomach, your soul, and every fiber of your being.

Let the words nurture you. Carry this book with you and open it to any page at any time of day for a message of hope and growth. This is the path to success: not just knowing, but living and believing, too.

While you read this book, allow yourself time to be completely focused. You may want to turn off the phone or lock the door or tell people that you will be unavailable for the next few hours. Give this time to yourself now so that you can find what you have been seeking for so long. This is your time.

As you take in these words, allow yourself to think new thoughts and find new visions. Keep a notebook at your side that can become your own personal journal of discovery. Underline or highlight the ideas in this book that resonate with you. You may want to play some relaxing music. Begin this journey knowing that your life is ready to bloom. You are ready to discover yourself in ways that may surprise you. When we open ourselves to change, we begin to learn from others, from nature, from our inner selves, and from the higher wisdom that fills our universe. Our own creativity and intuitive knowing begin to dance inside us, connecting us with other people and with spirit. Our hearts open wide and bring sunshine where there were only gray skies. Underneath the extra weight is so much beauty and self-fulfillment. Reducing weight will open the path toward the deeper peace that is waiting for us. Join me on the journey, hand in hand, heart in heart.

Fall in Love With Your Body

Conventional wisdom used to tell us that food was the only aspect to discovering the beautiful you. Today, we know that there's so much more—mental, physical and spiritual. Even though our senses tell us that the body is a solid, frozen, anatomical structure, fixed in space and time, this is not really the case. The truth is that our bodies are rivers of intelligence, information, and energy—constantly renewing themselves in every second of their existence. The body is not so much a "thing" as it is a process. Even with the physical, there are more aspects to your radiance than food alone. In this step, we'll focus on four areas that will help you reach your ideal weight:

- nourishing your body with food and drink
- moving your body
- resting your body
- nurturing your body through attention to your senses.

My key for discovering your body beautiful is moderation and balance. Moderate portions, balanced food groups, balancing food and movement, balancing your activities for others with nurturing for yourself, and balancing your interest in food with your interest in life.

A New Approach to Eating

Eating is paradoxical. It can give a sense of satisfaction, or it can leave us feeling empty. Haven't we all stared into an open refrigerator asking, "What do I want?" We may eat, whether we're hungry or not, only to discover that what we want is not in the refrigerator.

Eating when we're not hungry is a sign that food and our Inner Self are disconnected. We confuse our need for food with a need for other kinds of nourishment. Food can become a compensation for not having love. We may be instead starving from a lack of spiritual nourishment. We may be overwhelmed with emotions and eat food to calm and numb the feelings. We eat and eat, hoping it will somehow reach the part of ourselves that is truly in need of nourishment.

At the same time, we know so much about what to eat and what not to eat. Calories, kilos, carbohydrates, proteins, starvation diets, pineapple diets, yogurt diets...every month when the magazines arrive at the kiosk, we learn about a new miracle cure for our extra weight. Counting calories, watching the scale, and tracking diet plans may show short term success, but eventually the weight comes back. Some diet plans ask you to eat foods that are completely foreign to your lifestyle. Some tell you to eliminate certain food groups completely. You may be motivated to try any of these plans for a few weeks, but we always fall back into what's familiar. Completely depriving yourself of the foods you love is a recipe for failure.

We also know that if food isn't filling and nutritious, your body will scream for more. If you starve yourself with miniature portions, your body will automatically slow your metabolism and begin to conserve whatever energy you give it. When the diet is finished, the body quickly replenishes what it has lost. And you know what that means? It means you've just yo-yoed yourself!

How do we make sense out of this confusion? How do we learn to eat in a way that doesn't duplicate all the old habits and old thinking we've lived with for so long? We can no longer diet. We can no longer consider ourselves victims of our waistlines. No more battles. No more suffering.

When I was overweight, I never ate breakfast. I never really knew when I was hungry, and I never could tell when I was full. I ate when the clock said it was lunchtime or dinnertime. I ate portions that I thought were just right even though they left me feeling bloated and sleepy. I was always taught to clean my plate, so I never realized that I could eat a few bites of something and leave the rest. I had to let go of all this thinking and begin to be conscious of what my body truly needed.

As your body adjusts to your new food choices, you will begin to feel what your body needs to feel balanced and energized. Now I start my day with a little muesli and fruit. At lunch and dinner I eat as much as my *body* wants, not as much as I was served or as my plate would hold. I ask myself first how I feel instead of eating without being aware of this feeling. Thinking of myself first, instead of the food, keeps my priority clear. In this way, I respect my body and trust it to tell me what I really need.

When I first started teaching my weight loss courses, I wanted to tell people, "This program is not about food!" But no one would have believe me. How can a weight reduction course not be about food? They would have thought I was crazy.

I had heard a famous doctor, Dr. Michael Klaper, was coming to Switzerland. Though he was a cardiologist, he also had a program of healthy eating that helped his patients reduce their weight so they would have less strain on their hearts. I went to his lecture and afterward went to him for advice. "Dr. Klaper, we both know losing weight has more do with changing habits and thinking than it does with food. We know diets don't work. But people need guidelines. What do you tell your patients to eat?" We met for an hour or so and created what later became my formula for healthy eating. This formula has kept me at my ideal weight for 15 years. If you eat this way in conjunction with using the other ideas in this book, you, too, will reach your ideal weight.

An Uncomplicated Look at What to Eat

Are You Hungry for Food?

When you find yourself reaching for food, check in with your body and ask if you are really hungry for food. If your stomach is satisfied, ask your heart, "what do I really need?" It could be that you need to move your body or you need a nap. You may need to talk to a friend or spend some time alone. Ask your whole body…what is this impulse trying to tell me? Our bodies are our best friends. They give signals through feelings and emotions, and they also tell us when they have had enough.

If you are hungry for food, make a conscious decision about what you will eat. Some foods will make your body feel strong and balanced, while other foods will actually make you feel more hungry than before you ate them. We demand a lot from our bodies. Your body gets you up in the morning, walks, runs, lifts, bends, thinks, feels…what can you do for your body? Give it foods that will fuel it in the most efficient and energetic way. Give it good nutrition.

I made a decision to keep these food guidelines simple, and here's why: the more day-to-day energy you give to a problem, the bigger it gets. Have you ever been on a calorie-counting diet? I remember sitting in a restaurant with a calorie counter adding up the ingredient lists of each menu item before I could make a decision. That may seem a little silly, but it took so much energy to just get through each meal that I quickly lost interest in this method of eating. It wasn't practical, because by the time I added up all the lists and made my decision, it would be time to get back to work. Instead of feeling satisfied, I'd only feel frustrated.

Our bodies do a lot for us.

Giving food so much attention gives it a power that is out of step with the rest of your life. So instead of focusing on calories and grams, I want you to focus on eating **nutritious, whole foods in moderate amounts**.

Mary's Guidelines for Eating Every Day

Before you eat anything, ask yourself if you are really hungry for food.

When you are hungry, eat in moderation. Nothing is forbidden.

Choose each day:

- 3 handfuls of carbohydrates
- 5 fruits, either fresh or dried
- A little finger of fat
- 1 handful of protein
- All the vegetables you want
- Water

Three Handfuls of Carbohydrates

For sound nutrition, eat a handful of complex carbohydrates three times per day. Complex carbohydrates like rice, potatoes, bread, and polenta are all high in fiber, energy producing and easily processed by your body. Don't eat less than this. You need fuel to help you burn fuel. Instead of making your body bulge on the outside and clog up on the inside, these foods will fill you up, satisfy your body's nutritional demands, and keep your system running smoothly. Make complex carbohydrates a staple in your daily eating.

One Handful of Protein

Proteins like fish, meat, eggs, and nuts are an important part of nutrition, but we usually eat more protein than we actually need. One handful of a protein-packed food is enough for most people. Think also about how much fat is in the protein foods you choose. If you usually eat beef, pork, and lamb, think about alternating those meals with fish or chicken. If you choose not to eat meat, that's fine, too. Just be conscious of getting your protein from other sources.

Five Handfuls of Fruit

Fruits, either fresh or dried, give us instant energy with no fat. Years ago we didn't have the variety of fruit throughout the year. We stored apples in the cellar, and by March they were not very attractive, but we ate one or two. Now we have kiwi from Jakarta, mango from Hawaii, and clementines from Spain. Add fruit to your morning cereal, or squeeze a couple of oranges for a fresh glass of juice.

Vegetables, Vegetables, Vegetables

Vegetables, especially green vegetables, are packed with nutrition and are low in calories. Eat as much of these as you want. They'll satisfy your hunger and give you the vitamins and minerals you need to be healthy. Be creative with adding mushrooms, zucchini, eggplant to your usual sauces. Don't forget that fresh spices like basil, oregano, rosemary and tarragon are also healthy and add wonderful flavor.

A Finger of Fat A Day

Look at your little finger. Depending on your age, body, and activity level, that finger represents anywhere from 25 to 60 grams of fat. That's about how much fat you need in one day to be healthy. Now that may seem like a wide range. This is where you decide for yourself how much is too much. It's not the numbers that will help you reduce your weight—it's that you are taking responsibility for the effect it has on your body. The food you eat is your choice. You know you want to reduce your weight. You know that a finger of fat a day is all you need.

Just remember that, in the words of Dr. Michael Klaper, "The fat you eat is the fat you wear."

Cooking in non-stick pans, roasting food in the oven instead of frying, and using bouillon as a sauce base instead of cream or butter are all creative ways of cooking with less fat. Using less fat when you cook means you can have a finger of cheese of a piece of chocolate without guilt.

Water, Water Everywhere

Water is essential to a healthy body, and most of us don't drink enough. I try to drink at least eight glasses a day, either mineral water or still water—always with a twist of lemon or lime. Drink as much water as you have thirst for. It can help control your appetite and aid your digestion. As your body begins to lose fat, water also helps flush out the by products.

I used to drink water from any old cup I had around. Then one day I bought an elegant, crystal water glass and took it home. Suddenly, drinking water, which had been just a necessity, felt like a special event! I felt like royalty drinking from this beautiful glass. In my seminars, people often buy themselves a new water glass as a gift for taking their first step toward their ideal weight. Make water a special event. Use the most beautiful glass you have, or buy yourself a new one as a special present to yourself.

If you like coffee, tea, and sodas (as I do), be conscious of how much you're drinking. Coffee, tea, and soda are so pleasurable! However, the caffeine in coffee and tea can make some people jittery and can increase their appetite. The sugar in sodas can make them the equivalent of drinking a candy bar. Just be aware of what's in the food and drinks you're taking into your body.

When it comes to your choices, realize that nothing is forbidden! Even fat is not forbidden. You know that anything forbidden is just that much more attractive than something that isn't. Instead of telling yourself, "I can't have that," ask yourself, "what is possible for me today to eat?" All foods are possible. I am free to eat everything that follows my desires. Even chocolate. A spoonful of fat each day is just fine. Flexibility and moderation makes all foods possible. Be flexible instead of fanatic and you will find the path to a whole life. You can reach your ideal weight from your head down to your toes. You don't have to deprive yourself.

Have A New Relationship With an Orange

When I first started changing my eating habits, people told me to eat fruit as an alternative to something sweet. Fruit? "How boring," I thought. I remember as a little kid coming into the kitchen wanting a cookie and my mom occasionally saying, "Have an apple instead." Fruit, in my mind, was the poor substitute for what I really wanted but couldn't have.

As an adult, I realized that I still had this same notion planted in my head. So one day, I went to the grocery store and picked out the most beautiful orange I could find. I took it home, holding its round shape in my palm. I looked it over, smelled its rind, rubbed its nubby-smooth skin, and finally peeled it, very slowly. I ate each section slowly, savoring the burst of tart and sweet juice hitting my tongue.

This was not deprivation. This was a total food experience. From then on, I enjoyed having fruit as a snack or dessert without feeling in the least like I was eating what was second best.

Are there foods that you might want to become reacquainted with? Go to the store and choose the most beautiful one you can find. Don't just settle for any old apple. Choose the one that delights your eyes, nose, and touch, as well as your tastebuds.

Learn to cherish the foods that satisfy your intention for ideal weight. If you feel that what you're eating is only a replacement for what you'd rather be eating, you'll eventually binge and go back to your old habits. Your new food choices should fill you with joy because they are an important part of your new life. Give your tastebuds and body time to adjust, and if you're like me, all the foods that keep you at your ideal weight will taste like the most wonderful sensations in the world.

Care for Your Body

Movement is just as important as the food you choose. Making new choices about food is only part of the story. To keep your body healthy, you need to move. Any kind of movement is fine, as long as you do it. Do as much as you like. More is not always better, and a little is better than none. I love to walk outdoors in a beautiful setting, watching the seasons change. I also like to swim, and who doesn't love to dance in the living room? Find a way to move that makes you feel good—and don't forget to be thankful for the amazing miracle of your body.

Give your body adequate rest every day. Starving your body from sleep is another form of suffering that we can give up. Your mind and spirit will be refreshed and energized when your body is well rested. If you stay up late and have to get up early to go to work, try to take a short nap after you get home. Even if you lay down for 15 minutes, this can be precious rejuvenation time. In one or two weeks you and your body will be living together in comfort with mutual respect and love down to every cell.

Nurture Your Senses

The right food, water, and movement are good beginnings to a healthy body, but there's more our beings crave. We are holistic beings that take in every experience at a number of different levels, physical and non-physical. Our five senses all need "feeding," which helps stimulate our awareness and sense of balance. Our sixth sense, our higher self, needs feeding too.

We usually use our senses without thinking about them. When we see a beautiful tree, we usually don't think about how miraculous it is that we can see. We usually appreciate how beautiful the tree is. Self care helps us take time to appreciate our experience. We see the tree and we appreciate having the ability to see the tree. We notice the bright green of the leaves, and we also begin to notice the birds perched deep in the branches. We wonder how deep the roots must go to support such a large tree. We notice that the cloudy sky has passed and now the tree stands against a clear blue sky. We hear the wind in the leaves. The more aware we become, the more our senses are satisfied with our experience.

Notice how you are breathing, how your body moves with your breath. Someone walks by with a perfume, and you wonder what it is. You sit next to someone on the train, and your senses are filled with their presence. They are just like you…young or old, parents or children, all with a destiny. In these few minutes that your lives come together, you wonder about them, aware that you share your basic humanity with them. We are going to stimulate, love, and pamper all of our senses. This sparks our motivations. All of our senses begin to work together in perfect harmony. We discover that we are walking, living, breathing miracles.

Becoming more aware is a skill you can develop. Try once a day to slow down and focus on some aspect of self care. Here are some ideas to start with. Add your own ideas to the list, and then do them!

Eyes/Sight

- What's your favorite color? Buy a picture or a piece of clothing that reminds you of that color.
- Go outside and take a walk around your neighborhood. Look for ten things you've never noticed before.
- Put slices of cucumber on your closed eyes for a soothing sensation.

Nose/Smell

- Flower, flowers, flowers! Bring a fragrant bouquet into your house every week. Pick the flowers for their fragrance instead of their colors.
- Wear a new perfume.
- Use aromatherapy oils in your bath.
- Burn scented candles or incense in your home.

Skin/Hands/Touch

- Get a relaxation massage.
- Get a manicure and pedicure.
- Take a long, warm bath by candlelight.
- Scrub your skin gently all over with a dry loofah to stimulate circulation.
- After exercise, it feels especially good to give your skin extra attention. Indulge your body with a vitamin or mineral enriched lotion.

Ears/Hearing

- Listen to music you love but haven't heard for awhile or ever before.
- Turn the radio on to a station you don't know and listen.
- Go outside and concentrate on the sounds you hear. How many things can you hear? Birds? Cars? Voices? Leaves and grass rustling in the wind? Doors opening?
- Listen to love songs and fall in love with the music. Or listen to rock and roll songs, sing along, and dance with yourself.
- Ask someone close to you to tell you, "I love you." Listen closely.

Learn to Observe Yourself

As you become more intimate with yourself, learn to observe your actions without judgement. For example, do you really know what you eat? Are you aware of every bite that goes into your mouth? "Of course," you might be thinking.

When I was raising three little boys I spent a lot of time in the kitchen. I cooked three meals a day, made snacks, and cooked for friends and neighbors who would come for dinner. I was always over-weight, and I couldn't really understand why, because at meals I ate very little.

One day my friend Marilyn was over, and I told her how frustrated I was with this. "I can't understand why I'm fat. I don't eat that much!"

Marilyn looked at me closely. Then she said, "Mary, maybe you eat more than you realize."

What? I didn't know what I was eating? That seemed ridiculous. And even though I was a little hurt that she would say this to me, I knew she was trying to tell me something I needed to hear, so I listened.

She said, "I've noticed that when you clear up the table, you finish the last bites off the boys' plates, and when you're dishing up ice cream for them, you take bites for yourself. And when you bake, you're always taking bites. I know you think of it as tasting, but it's still food, and it's still going into your body, and it still counts."

Did I really do those things? I couldn't even picture myself doing those things. I wondered if she was making this up.

In the coming days I made a decision to watch my eating—not to change it, just to observe it with new eyes. And you know what? Marilyn was right. All those extra bites were usually in the midst of stress. I would be talking on the phone, or calling for the boys, or jug-gling six plates on their way to the table, but all the while I was slipping in bites here and there.

Because my attention was undirected, I didn't even notice that I was eating those extra bites. I was completely unaware of my own habits, and until Marilyn told me the truth, I denied that I had those habits. Suddenly I knew where those extra kilos came from.

I thought about the frenzy of activity that kept my attention away from my eating and automatically moved my hand to my mouth without so much as a thought. I asked myself why I had to eat in the midst of this whirlwind. And the answer I heard from inside was, "Mary, you're frustrated."

The hardest part was admitting that I was in denial about my eating. Was I really so unconscious of my own habits? Was I really so out of touch with my own behavior that I wasn't even aware of the food that was going in my mouth? I had to admit that I was afraid of my eating problem. I had to face myself honestly. Acknowledging that fear, though, allowed me to let it go and move to a place where I could take action to change.

Even if you think you are entirely aware of your eating habits, it can be enlightening to observe your own habits for several days in a row. Don't try to change your patterns. And please, please don't judge yourself. Just watch and learn about yourself.

The point is to see yourself in a new light. The point is to reveal new information about your habits that will help you understand better what you need. Recognizing these underlying patterns is one of the keys to permanent weight reduction. It is also critical to realizing what you really want in your life instead of the extra food.

When you see how you really act, instead of how you think you should act, you can begin to make realistic intentions and beliefs to support your transition from behavior that limits you toward behavior that supports you.

Ideal Weight and Your Infinite Possibility

Even though our senses tell us that the body is a solid, frozen, anatomical structure, fixed in space and time, this is not really the case. The truth is that our bodies are rivers of intelligence, information, and energy—constantly renewing themselves in every second of their existence. The body is not so much a "thing" as it is a *process*.

That process is affected by our habits and the choices we make each day. Our bodies are carrying out tasks for us non stop the whole day and often on into the night. There doesn't seem to be enough time in the day to do all that we think we have to do. We do everything for everyone else making deadlines, taking care of families, cooking the meals, cleaning, and working. "I don't have time," we say, and it becomes the excuse for not taking care of ourselves. The eventual result, when we don't nurture ourselves, is stress and tiredness. We have always been rewarded for doing more and more, until stress tells us it's time to stop. We know that over time stress causes our blood pressure to rise, can bring on headaches, or even heart problems.

Our old way of compensation was eating. But now that we are more aware of the ways we can nurture our bodies—with rest, attention to our senses, nutritious food, clear water. Too much food only makes the stress worse and blocks the path to light and love. Your intention, your heart's desire, is to give positive regard to your body, not to betray yourself.

Appeal to your higher self, the part of you that gives you love, your soul. Cry out to the highest part of your self and ask for guidance. Take deep breaths. Sit quietly. Trust your intuition. Ask your heart, "what does my body really need?"

You have time for you. Take yourself to the door and go for a walk. Push against your resistance to get through to the other side of yourself, the side that cares for you. Intimacy with the Self brings about true healing.

Discovering this caring part of you is a form of intimacy with the Self. Like meeting a new friend, this part of you cares about how you feel. This is the path to self love. When you truly find this love, you find yourself. You find acceptance and your dreams and desires.

Reaching the *body* of your heart's desire is not just about *food*. Food choices are important, but that is only one component in the path to ideal weight.

You are More Than What You Think

Thinking with symbols gives us power to jump out of old thought patterns. Think of the process of bringing new ideas into your life like breaking in a new pair of shoes. The new shoes are clean, beautiful, and in perfect condition. But they're not as comfortable as the old, well-worn pair. Sometimes the new shoes pinch a little.

So you wear the new shoes when you go out, and you love how they look, but you don't always love how they feel. When you get home, you put the Old Shoes on because their fit is so familiar. The new shoes may give you pleasure, but they still aren't the ones you reach for when you want comfort.

However, you don't stop trying to get used to the new shoes, because they are beautiful. The old pair is simply worn out, and you're ready for a new change.

After a couple of weeks, the new shoes get broken in, and they feel more comfortable. Before long you forget that they were a bit tight at first, and when you catch your reflection in a mirror or shop window you smile. You like them now, and they've become comfortable.

Once in awhile you see the old pair in the bottom of your closet, and occasionally you put them on again. But they don't feel right anymore. They look worn out and faded. You've changed, and they no longer fit

changing habits

with the person you have become. Eventually you throw them out, because you know you'll never wear them again.

Your old ideas about food are an old pair of shoes. At this point, if you're like most people in my seminars, you've committed yourself halfway to the dream of your ideal weight. You may still have doubts, or you still remember all those other times you tried to lose weight and ended up losing your courage.

So how do we turn that half commitment into full-hearted enthusiasm? Let's explore what's going on inside our minds that either helps or hinders our ability to fall in love with our new shoes—our new bodies and our whole self.

"Negative" Emotions Are Messages from Inside

Some people say all behavior is either an act of love or a cry for help. The acts of love fill us with joy and pride. They surround us with a glow that uplifts the people around us.

There is also frustration, disappointment and confusion. We've all felt them. Maybe we've been eating over them for years. We usually want to get away from them as fast as possible, sometimes at any cost, because we want only comfort.

But let's take a look at these three emotions in another light. Frustration, disappointment and confusion are just as essential to growth as are joy, pride and happiness. These emotions, through the pain they cause us, strongly stimulate us to change and learn. They are an indication that we are moving into a new awareness. If we move with their lessons, their presence is only temporary. When we resist their lessons, we spiral downward.

Emotions are messages. Frustration, disappointment and confusion are part of the human experience. You can deny them, hide from them and refuse to admit that they have a message for you. But I want to give you some new ideas about these emotions so that you can begin to understand their messages. As you read these next passages, you might remember situations where you felt these emotions. Write those thoughts down if your like. Your insights and ideas are important!

Frustration

Have you ever misplaced your keys? Remember rummaging through the house knowing they're so very near but completely out of reach! If you did this repeatedly, you probably found a system to make sure you always have your keys in the same place.

I'm sure you know the frustration of trying to lose weight. Frustration is probably part of the reason you decided to pick up this book, right? In the past, that frustration could have led you to the kitchen cupboards or to another serving of food you didn't need. Unfortunately, that response kept you rooted in the problem, becoming even more frustrated than you were before!

But your response this time—to recommit yourself to reaching your ideal weight—transforms your frustration into emotional fuel for positive action. I remember the exact moment when I finally decided to let go of my extra weight. I wasn't feeling good that day. In fact, I was pretty depressed! I was thinking, "I'm sick and tired of being fat, and I won't put up with it anymore!" That was the point that I knew I had had enough. My frustration level couldn't get any higher, and I decided that the only solution was to *make a different response to my problem.*

Now, think about that for a moment. What we think of as a negative emotion gave me the energy and motivation to make a positive change! Maybe it's the same for you. If you weren't frustrated, you wouldn't care about making a change.

reframing

Confusion

Confusion...it feels like you can't see a thing clearly, you have no clue about how you're going to get through, and sometimes you wonder if you'll even get through at all.

Confusion can make you feel panic and unsettled. Everything seems so mixed up. Nothing is the same as it was. You feel like your brain is a mixed salad of disoriented thoughts. But as your brain frantically sorts for answers and patterns that give meaning to your new experience, your mind opens up to ideas that could never before find space. Go back silently to ask your heart, "What do I really want?" Then listen. It really works, every time.

Disappointment

If you have expectations, you have experienced disappointment. When you dream a dream, there's always the possibility that it won't come true exactly as you expected.

That thought alone is enough to stop some people from going one step further. If there's a possibility of failure, then why even try? Why indeed? Because nothing was ever gained without taking a risk.

Taking a risk doesn't mean leaping out of an airplane without a parachute or climbing a mountain without the right shoes. Taking a risk does mean being willing to step out of your comfort zone, to go exploring with an open heart and a willingness to accept what you find.

In order to live your dreams, you have to be *willing* to step into the new shoes. You have to be *willing* to put the old memory on hold, even though you don't immediately have a new memory to replace it. You have to be *willing* to step into the space between the old habits and the new habits, secure in the fact that you will be given what you need to get to the new place you want to be. Have faith and trust in your all-knowing self.

You have to be willing to look at each step along the way as a triumph of courage, no matter what you find in that new territory. But first you have to choose to take that risk, and when you do, that openness of spirit will carry you the whole way.

Guilt

Guilt is about regret. Guilt is about an action or feeling that you wish were different than it is. Maybe you believe that you should feel differently than you do. Maybe you believe you should be different than you are. You sense that you've gone against your own standards. You feel that these changes are in your power but somehow beyond your reach. Guilt can be so very depressing, but think about this: if you didn't have a sense of your own values and the values of those you care about, you couldn't feel guilt. And this awareness of values is a positive thing in our lives. Experiencing guilt, at one level, is a sign that you are in touch with what you believe.

When we were children, our parents gave us beliefs that we should act in a certain way, and this guided our behavior and molded who we have become. As adults, we can re-evaluate those beliefs to bring them in line more closely with our own intentions. I no longer believe that I "should" eat everything on my plate in order to be healthy. I no longer believe that I "should not" have a career.

When I gave up these beliefs, I felt some guilt, not because I didn't believe wholeheartedly in my new thoughts but because they were in conflict with certain things my mother taught me. What I had to accept is that I can have my own unique beliefs without betraying the love of those around me.

What I discovered is that I can care about someone else without adopting their beliefs! This is one of the keys to letting go of guilt forever. The other solution to letting go of guilt is forgiveness. We often find it easier to forgive other people for mistakes than to forgive ourselves. It's so easy to occupy ourselves with obsessive thoughts about "What I should have done..." Instead, accept that you are in the process of growth, and that process takes time. A flower doesn't go from seed to full bloom in a day. You are a flower that needs care and nurturing. Forgive yourself, accept that mistakes are an opportunity for learning, and move on.

You can envision yourself guilt-free in the same way that you can see yourself thin. First, think about something that makes you feel guilty. Imagine it as a lead coat that hangs on you, pulling your shoulders down, pushing in your chest so you can't breathe, constricting your arms and legs from moving freely. Can you feel it? Can you feel the tremendous weight of it all?

Now, relax your shoulders and feel the coat sliding off your body onto the ground. Let it be there. You don't have to move it ever again. You never have to wear that coat again. Do you feel lighter? Let the Earth take the coat back, because you don't need that feeling anymore.

Guilt, like pain, can either pull you down into a quicksand of negative feelings, or it can be a tool for learning and growth. Recognize your feelings, but remember that they are really just a warning light that something in your value system and daily steps needs to be explored. Make a decision to bring what you need into your life—love, self acceptance, perseverance—and to let go of the guilty feelings that only keep you down.

Shame

Feelings of shame can permeate every corner of life. It's a veil through which the world looks darker, sadder and more threatening. A shame-based way of thinking can begin early in life when a child is given the message that he or she is not fully accepted or does not fully meet the standards of family and friends. That child may begin to think, "I'm not good enough," or, "I'm a mistake." This feeling, coming from the outside, takes root inside. That message is triggered every time the child makes a mistake.

Once a child links ordinary mistakes with a deep sense of shame, learning stops. Would you be willing to take a risk if you knew that even a small mistake would feel devastating to you? Shame shifts the focus from even the greatest success back to failure. Even the smallest mistake is seen as an indication of inadequacy. Those small problems trigger memories of larger issues of shame, and a cycle is formed.

Gina, a woman in my seminar, remembers being eight years old and shopping for school clothes with her sister and mother. She and her mother were both overweight, while her ten-year-old sister was not. Gina loves the color red, but her mother never let her buy anything vibrant or bright. Her mother would choose subdued blues or browns from the clothes racks, holding them up saying, "This will help you not be noticed…" Meanwhile, the sister was dressed out in brilliant, eye-catching colors.

While the mother's positive intention in selecting those clothes was to shield her daughter from being noticed and teased about her weight, she in fact taught Gina a different lesson: if you're fat, your body is disgusting to other people, so you should try not to be seen. Even after Gina lost weight in her adult life and started to wear all her favorite bright colors, she still found herself feeling uncomfortable when anyone commented on her new clothes.

Shame really means that you don't feel whole and worthy of love from other people. Shame makes us feel vulnerable and unloved. Shame buries your authentic, powerful self. The part that is most unique and true about a person becomes a hidden, unknown mystery and disconnects from our spirit. Sometimes a wall of fat will lessen that pain by placing a barrier between us and the people we feel rejected by. This is a very real protection, but when we block out pain we also block out the potential for love. The very fear of intimacy prevents it.

No one can ever see the real you if you are hiding behind your extra weight. Paradoxically, shame can also make us feel small inside, like we have no substance. Extra weight can make us feel substantial again. Extra physical size, in some sense, is used to compensate for a diminished sense of self.

Fear

Our biggest block in finding and developing ourselves is fear. The last thing we want to do is feel our fears. We often do everything we can do avoid them. I believe fear stops us for only one reason: so we will look at it. Fear has a message for us.

One of the most common fear is **fear of the unknown**. Fear reminds us that we can't control every outcome, and we can't know the future. We can plan and act with conscious attention, but the future is a combination of our own actions and what the universe brings to us. Perfect control is an illusion. When we were kids just learning about the world, *everything* was unknown, and still we pushed on and explored. The fact that you're here says that you are willing to accept change and the uncertain feelings that may come with it. That is an important step. Give yourself a hand for being so open, and promise yourself that it's only one of many moments that you will find the wisdom, courage, faith and trust that keeps you on a path of love instead of a path of fear. Accept each step.

Another fear that is part of the human experience is the **fear of loss**. We fear losing what we know. We fear losing what makes us feel safe and secure. Even when we don't like an old habit, it's like that old comfortable shoe. It doesn't fit anymore, but when you throw it out, it's a loss.

We are going to be afraid from time to time. Buddhist Pema Chödrön says that *fear is a natural reaction to moving closer to the truth.* If you are on a path of truth for yourself, you will face fear. As we learn, change and develop we encounter unknown waters like a ship going to its destination. Some days are smooth sailing, then suddenly comes a storm. Does the ship turn back to its safe harbor? Or does the ship sail on? Sometimes we can't face our fear, and we go back to old ways. Other times we find the courage to go on. Every situation brings with it the seeds of a new opportunity to learn to handle our fears, facing them directly and honestly.

As we become more intimate with our fears, we learn that *fear is always about the future*. We don't have anxiety about the past because the past is gone. We lived through our unknown fears of the past. We do, however have memories of the past. We have our regrets and our solutions from the past. We wish we would have done some things better. Other times we were surprised at how well we found solutions. We have mixed feelings about the past. We're guilty about the things we wish we had done better and thankful about the things we did well. Our memories and pain from the past ignite new feelings about the future.

When we live in fear, our emotions run us in a circle: old pain from our old feelings reminds us of our old judgements of ourselves. We feel drained of courage, feel all our fear, and feel overwhelmed. In that state, we compensate ourselves with food or other distractions, which makes us feel the old pain all over again.

The truth is, you really can't lose anything. Everything transforms. Everything that changes becomes something else. The losses you suffer are a way to learn. Remember, fear is usually an illusion about something that hasn't even happened, and 92% of all the fears and worries we conjure up in our mind don't happen. But believe me, I know the *pain* of fear is always real, whether or not it ever comes true.

While in the midst of this vicious circle, I came one day to the notion that I could step into a different territory. Instead of being caught up in the emotions, I wondered if there was another viewpoint where I could feel grounded. Perhaps there is a *stillpoint* where I could face my fears without feeling that my very being was threatened by it.

I knew with relaxation I could find this space. Relaxing with my fear, I could look at it and feel it. Then I could make a decision to let it go. I didn't learn that growing up. What I learned in my past was to keep myself busy. I denied the awareness of fear with more and more work. Like a snowball gathering momentum as it rolls down a hillside, rampant productivity would overrun any message fear might be trying to send me. But the very activity that was fighting with the fear was itself out of control. Working too much, eating too much, smoking too much. It was all out of control.

What I needed to find was a stillpoint where all emotions are accepted as being part of the human process. Fear, sadness, disappointment, hope, joy, ecstasy—all are a part of development. From this point of acceptance and stability within ourselves, we can learn to be flexible with our emotions. We can observe that fear gives way to courage. Disappointment gives way to hope. Joy gives way to ecstasy. Ecstasy gives way to quiet satisfaction. Accepting that, we can begin to accept all of our emotions and enjoy their dance through our life.

To find this stillpoint and gain this acceptance of my emotions. Becoming still is not the same as being lazy. Stillness is calm and quiet—a state in which we can hear the voice from our higher consciousness.

Instead of living in a never ending circle of fear, we can learn to live in a circle of transformation: by letting go of the old pain, we begin to stay in the present. When we are in the present, we remember what it is we really want. We are able to listen to our inner, higher self. We walk in the new shoes, feel all our feelings and accept them. When those feelings bring up old pain, we let it go, completing the circle of transformation.

So now we have to learn to find the stillpoint inside. Not only do we have to stop and relax, meditate, listen to music, walk in the forest, but we also have to acknowledge all the feelings we have. When we pay attention to them, we bring their cries to consciousness. Not feeling our feelings can drive us once again in the direction of compulsive thinking and compulsive eating. When we allow ourselves to relax in silence, our thinking opens and we let go of what blocks us. We are not escaping our emotions. We are embracing them, because they are a part of the precious beauty within ourselves. There we find all the answers.

Whatever We Intend and Give Attention to, We Become

The faster your life is changing, the more difficult it may feel to stay on your path. By making a decision to change old habits, you ask the underlying causes of those habits to rise to the surface of your life. Right now you're accelerating the process of change in your life as you come closer to your ideal weight.

To stay on your path, you can consciously redirect your thinking to your heart, a simple step that will raise your spirits and bring back the truth: that you are love, that you are you, that negativity is not your destiny.

One way to change our thinking is to observe others without judgement. Observe others who have a sense of inner serenity, and you see what they know: life is a step by step process. They give themselves time to nurture new awareness and learn new things. They let solutions emerge from their bodies and minds—solutions that were learned through change, curiosity, and determination. They know patience. They know that when flowers are tiny seeds it sometimes takes months before they are brilliant and fully bloomed.

You know now that your reality is based on your intention. Carol was a client of mine who at one time was completely addicted to chocolate. She was easily influenced by what other people thought of her, especially when they were critical. Anytime someone criticized her, she immediately felt a deep sense of low self worth, and she would binge.

Carol successfully stopped this behavior by finding a new intention. She decided that if she was going to take control of her eating, she would have to find a new way to respond to criticism.

Think about a blooming plant that you might have. Imagine that one day you leave it in your backyard for some sunshine. The phone rings and you run inside to talk to your friend who's calling to tell you about what a fabulous day it's been. You forget about the plant, and later a strong storm comes up that breaks off the buds and fills the pot with water. You go outside after the storm and look up at the clearing sky. You look down, and there is your plant looking battered. You realize that you forgot about the plant. You blame yourself. Meanwhile, your drooping little plant just wants you to prop it up a little and give it some care and attention. Focusing on the mistake doesn't bring the plant back.

If you tend to be forgetful, figure out a way to help yourself remember. If you just plain made a mistake, repair the damage, forgive yourself and move on. It's important to learn from situations, but dwelling on them, avoiding responsibility, or giving attention to the negative side only keeps you trapped in behaviors that take you away from your vision.

When you find yourself reacting in a negative way:

1. Stop reacting. Be still, breathe deeply.
2. Ask your heart for a solution.
3. Sleep on it for three nights.
4. Be willing to accept the solution when it appears.

The last step may be more challenging than it seems. The path of heart is not always the most obvious or the one that makes the most "sense" to us. But your heart's answer is a true answer! Listen to it, accept it, and learn from it.

When something happens in your life that fills you with emotion, ask yourself, *"What does this mean for me?"* Your meaning of an event determines how you will feel about it. The answers to your questions will tell you whether you're viewing the event with a negative or positive attitude. Are your thoughts filled with words like "can't" and "won't" or are you asking "why" and "where" and "how"? Go back to being the observer. Observe the answers that come to you. Also observe your process of change.

Positive thinking does not live life looking through rose-colored glasses. A positive attitude doesn't deny that painful, difficult, tragic situations sometimes happen. A positive attitude doesn't deny that sometimes life doesn't seem fair. A positive attitude does mean that you approach life looking for ways to learn about yourself by asking questions, being curious and open to new answers instead of relying on old, habitual thinking.

When you think and talk positively, the gift of opportunity in every moment becomes more clear. You and the world are changing every single second. Negative thinking slows down your ability to use that change to make your life more full, more beautiful. Just as you have a choice to wear the new shoes today, you have a choice about what you think and what you say. You can choose every day.

Look Inside for Your Truth

The most important part of asking for answer from our Inner Selves is simply to ask. There is no right or wrong way to meditate or silence our minds so that the answer will come. Every way is a possible path to our own hearts. I wish I could give you a clear idea about how this process works, but it's like trying to explain how it feels to be in love. The words are only approximations. The experience develops like learning to love the smell of warm bread. Here is my process.

1. Find a place where you can be alone, with no distractions. Turn the phone answering machine on and the bell off. Make a promise to yourself not to answer the doorbell if it rings. This is your time.
2. Sit or lay down in a comfortable position.

3. Notice your breathing. Mentally observe the rising and falling of your chest. Notice the rhythm of your breaths, whether they are full or shallow. Observe your breathing. Just quietly notice it.

4. If you notice other sounds—footsteps on the sidewalk outside, birds at your window, cars passing on the street—just passively notice them and return your attention to your breathing.

5. As thoughts and feelings come into your mind, observe them as passively as you can. Things that normally might upset you are very far away. You don't have to solve or plan or react to any of these thoughts. You can see all these flickering thoughts with acceptance and equality.

6. Notice if your body is tense or relaxed. Start with your face and notice if your muscles are loose or tight. If they're tight, take a deep breath and imagine the tension melting away. One by one, notice your neck, arms, hands, chest, stomach, legs, and feet in the same way. If the tension won't go, don't worry. Just notice it and turn your attention back to your breath.

7. As thoughts come into your mind, let them flow through without judgement. Allow your thoughts to come and go. When a thought enters, notice it, then let it leave your mind. Just let the thoughts flow.

Try this for 20 minutes once a day. This process develops over time. When you try this, don't expect to do it all on the first try.

Meditation helps us detach from our emotions so that we can observe them and learn from them in a new way. The key is observing without judgement. Sitting still and quiet for even ten minutes brings into sharp contrast how busy we are the rest of our lives. By sitting in silence, we can begin to enter the stillpoint where the most important voice is heard—that of our own hearts.

This inner process will be different each time you do it. That's perfectly natural. You're not doing this for a certain outcome or result. In fact, you're simply making a space where inspiration and answers you didn't even know you were looking for can emerge. The messages your Inner Self sends you may be in the form of words, images, sounds, feelings, ideas…whatever their form, they come from the wise place inside you that holds all your answers. Be curious about your thoughts and the messages they hold.

Meditation has helped me to feel the deep connections between myself and other people, myself and the world. If everything in this world has a purpose, then that means I have a purpose, too—and so do you. Meditation opened the awareness that what I've been seeking all my life outside me really begins inside me.

When you do this practice for some time, your heart opens in new ways. A gentle strength enters you, and things you feared before don't seem to bother you anymore.

As I learned to do meditation I was at first trying to avoid pain, disappointments, and discouragement. Basically, unknown to myself, I had secretly hoped that if I did the practice I wouldn't have to feel pain anymore. That was certainly an illusion, because pain is a part of experiencing life. Meditation invites the pain in so you can see it in the same light that you see pleasure. Without judgment, without pushing it away, all experience becomes a part of being alive—a blessing, even when it seems to hurt.

The Seeds of Thought We Plant Will Grow

Whether negative talk is directed at yourself or someone else, it leads only to depression and despair. You've heard this before:

"I can't."

"It's not possible."

"This won't work."

"I always fail."

"I always gain the weight back."

The thoughts we plant in our bodies and minds can be beautiful and nourishing or they can be weeds that will eventually grow up around us and choke us. The only possible results of negative talk are no motivation, no success, no weight reduction, no rewards, and no self-esteem. What we intend to become, we will become. What we give attention to grows and develops.

Focus on Your Positive Possibilities

Every morning before I get out of bed, I take a few minutes to think about my day. I might have a day packed full of activities, which I know may be stressful, or I might have a quiet day all to myself. No matter what, I start the day by renewing my vision of whole body wellness and ideal weight. This daily ritual keeps the rest of my day centered.

Every day, ask yourself these questions:

"Do I want to stay in the my old habits or learn a new way of living?"

"How do I want to feel when I go to bed tonight?"

How you answer these questions is entirely up to you. Some days you may decide not to take a step toward your dream. Give yourself permission for that too. Please forgive yourself for not being perfect. Whatever your answer, let it be your conscious decision.

If you find yourself concentrating on what you can't eat, turn your ideas around. Think about what you can eat.

At one time I was in a serious car accident and lived in a wheelchair for an entire year. I was a single mom at the time and struggled with the reality that I could barely take care of my three boys. I couldn't work, so I was worried about money. My self-esteem was on the floor, I felt so helpless! There was nothing I could do. I felt trapped.

One day I was watching TV (I could at least do that), and an ad came on for the Open University in Houston. I had always wanted to get my college degree but had never been able to find the time or energy to do it. Well, now, what else could I do in a wheelchair except use my mind?

My body was broken. I called a friend and asked her if she would help me register. She came right over, wheeled me out the door, and I was on my way to a college career! For the next few months I was full of fear and wondered at times what I had gotten myself into! But taking that first step was the key.

There is opportunity in every situation. There is always something to be learned! I was in a deep depression when I made the decision to try college. I was desperate. I knew I had to do something to change the course of my life, or I would end up with a paralyzed mind, even after the casts came off my legs!

You may feel just as desperate about being overweight. But there is a wealth of new experiences waiting for you to discover them.

Rebuilding Life From a Universe of Infinite Possibility

When I redecorate a room, I go to all sorts of stores looking for ideas in color, pattern and texture. I look through tons of magazines and consider so many color schemes that you'd think I was decorating a palace instead of just one room. I confuse myself with all the possibilities, looking with fresh eyes at new color combinations that I never really looked at in quite the same way before. I do this because it shakes me out of my usual world and forces me to consider my problem in a new way.

And I'm always surprised at the outcome. Somewhere along the way, I make a discovery that takes me into a new way of seeing the room. It could be a new way of combining colors or a texture that I never thought I liked before but now feels oddly comforting.

Those moments of discovery, whether they're about decorating a room or seeing your life in a new way, don't come out of cool, logical thinking, and you can't get them out of a book. They only come when all that you know is thrown up in the air, and you work to find a new sense of order to it all.

What happens when we're hurting? Our heads go down, we look at the floor. Our vision turns away from the world into our pain. This is when we can lose sight of the horizon of our intention.

So lift your head up! Keep your faith in yourself by giving attention to your intention. Remember the vision of how you look and feel at your ideal weight. You may wonder if the actions you're taking and the thoughts you're having are going to make any difference to your life. You may feel like there's a lot you don't understand any more. You may feel sad because events outside you are not yet matching what you want inside. All these feelings are temporary.

If you're having doubts, make a decision to stop questioning yourself and simply follow through on your earlier intentions. The results will show themselves, but like the watched kettle that never boils, you will slow down your progress by expecting too much too soon.

If you feel confusion, ask yourself what you still understand clearly. Ask yourself what you know to be true. For example, you know that feeling confused is a normal part of the process of growth. You know that asking questions and allowing yourself to work through to the answers will take you to a place of personal understanding that will be healthy and emotionally uplifting.

You know that you are taking positive action every day. You know that you have all the resources available to support your transition. And you know that you will find the answers you need.

If you feel disappointment, let yourself feel the sadness of that. You may have to grieve an old expectation or intention that no longer fits with your life. If you overeat, you may feel sad that you slipped into the Old Shoes, even after you decided that you wouldn't ever do that again. You may feel sad that you've spent so many years away from your dreams. Let yourself feel that fully, observe it, and then *let it go*. Did someone else cause you disappointment? Learn what you can from this, and then slowly begin to let it go, step by step.

After you feel strong again, ask yourself what triggered these emotions. Notice how you reacted. Were you able to stick to your intention, even in the midst of the emotional storm? Just observe yourself and try to hear the message your inner self is sending. The message may feel negative and confusing. Keep asking your inner self what this means and what you need to do for yourself to bring your being into clarity and light.

Sometimes when we are moving toward what we value most, we find ourselves taking one step forward and one step back. This is called approach/avoidance. In other words, we begin moving toward our intention because we know it will bring us pleasure, but on the way we become afraid. The fear distracts us and throws us off our path. This fear can short-circuit feelings of motivation and our intention to act positively. We avoid facing the fear, and that prevents us from reaching our intention.

You can turn the fear around by giving attention to what is important to you…your vision. When you feel fear taking you toward the refrigerator, STOP. Take one minute—60 seconds—to renew your intention:

> *I am relentless about making my vision a reality.*
> *I am ready to change.*
> *I am responsible for my state of mind.*
> *Today I learn what I can, and I let go of the rest.*
> *I will find the answers I seek.*
> *I am a visionary in action, transcending my history in every way that is important to me.*
> *I have all I need inside myself to be successful now.*
> *I am free to choose what I eat today.*

It's absolutely essential that you allow yourself to feel all the feelings that come up about your weight and your life. Even if the feelings that come up are uncomfortable, you can use these emotions to give you emotional energy to decide what you really want out of life.

Remember that frustration, disappointment and confusion are signs that you are ready to change! These feelings may be just the things you need to make the decision that you will absolutely not tolerate being overweight any longer. Now start by standing in front of a mirror and saying out loud,

"I will no longer tolerate being overweight."

Say it again, louder,

"I will no longer tolerate being overweight!"

Shout it at the top of your lungs if necessary until you are clear with yourself.

The Pleasure Principle

When is your body feeling at its best? The answer is simple, when you are happy. Why do you end up carrying too much weight? Can it be true that we are weighed down not only by kilos but also by our unhappiness? Have we made our unhappiness a habit?

As seekers of our highest selves we now go toward lightness instead of darkness. It is a wonderful symbol, because in reality our spirits are higher on a sunny day than on a dark, rainy day. We seek pleasure on a sunny day, while we usually stay inside on a rainy day. In darkness, we hide from the pleasure that is ours to enjoy.

You have a dream of reaching your ideal weight, and I believe that experiencing more pleasure will get you there faster. What most people do is avoid pleasure and punish themselves for being overweight. We go into the closet, so to speak. We don't move our bodies because we are uncomfortable with the way we look. We don't walk on the beach because we hate the way we look in a bathing suit. So instead of pleasure, you sit in the dark with guilt or shame…punishing yourself with the very thing that makes you fat. Those of us who have been over-weight all know this vicious circle.

Let us break out of these old patterns that have caused us to spiral downward. Instead, let's try a whole new system that begins with giving attention to pleasure. What we give attention to expands. That means when we give attention to punishing ourselves, we punish and punish and punish. No pleasure is allowed. We don't even give ourselves the pleasure of eating.

Now we are going to *enjoy* everything we eat. Eating the things that please you in moderation is wiser than giving yourself pain with dieting. Believe that you are not suffering, and you will find the freedom to give yourself pleasure. Giving pleasure is connected with the love you are developing with your higher self. Pleasure raises your Spirits.

You don't deserve to punish yourself ever again. You can give up suffering. Is suffering a choice? Sure it is! If we know we cause every situation, every experience that happens to us, then we are going to be the conductors of our own music…the orchestrators of our own lives. You have felt cheated and angry about not being able to enjoy life. Now we are going to turn that around.

Try some of these ideas:

- Make a date with yourself. Go to a movie in the middle of the day, and out for coffee afterward.
- Have your astrology chart done. It's really fun!
- Do something creative that you have always wanted to do. It is amazing how involved you can get with something like taking a watercolor course. Make a deal with your partner that you have one night out for your creativity.
- Try a new look, get a new hair cut or makeover.
- Learn something new. Take a computer course. You may be surprised by how much fun it can be.

- Go to a play or a concert.
- Take dance lessons or yoga lessons.

Do all of this for fun, just for you, remembering all the time that **you deserve all the love and pleasure that you can give yourself.**

Reaching your own ideal weight automatically gives you more pleasure. Now you can allow even more pleasure every day. You are going to put yourself in an important position in your life. You are number one. I know you have felt less important than other people, for instance other members of your family. Yet we all know that when we are not happy, our families are miserable. The best thing we can do for others is learn to be happy with ourselves. When we love ourselves, we have love to give others.

Fall in Love With Spirit

Every moment holds the possibility of change. The chance to transform ourselves into beings of greater love and happiness is always hovering near us. We learn lessons every day. Some are new. Other lessons are familiar but perhaps we haven't learn them well enough. They again arrive on our doorsteps asking to be further developed and transformed. We are on a path of enlightenment.

Right at this moment, we are changing. It's an inescapable truth. Our bodies and thoughts change moment by moment. Our bodies renew themselves. Skin sheds itself. Hair falls out and grows again. Fingernails grow, get cut, and grow again. New wrinkles appear. We get older, but our bodies continue to renew themselves. In a very real way, I am not the same body that first created and taught *Für Immer Schlank*, my weight loss course in Switzerland, eight years ago.

Change happens in our inner beings just as it happens in our outer bodies. We are thinking and feeling beings, capable of deciding our future and making decisions about how to live inside our bodies. Do we want a healthy body? Or do we want to use our body as a block to our happiness? It's a choice that comes from our conscious thought and manifests itself in our cells. What we see in the mirror isn't just our physical being. We also see an image of our inner self. We are the reflection of our inner self.

We are each an individual capable of choice. We are also members of families, a town, a country, and a culture. It's only natural to be aware of what others think of us. This is a given part of being interrelated. Those opinions sometimes synchronize with our inner knowing, but sometimes they drown out what we know is best for us. When the outer voices are louder than the inner voice of wisdom, we may give up on our own path to satisfy others. "This is what my parents say is best for me. This is what my culture tells me is right. This is what my friends say I should do. And they all know better than I do." Looking to others for answers is a way of seeking comfort, but what we receive from others doesn't always fit who we are. We are seeking our own Soul, a higher awareness that leads us to peace and happiness.

Referring always to others can't bring us happiness. Trying to satisfy everyone else while leaving our own desires in the background only makes us frustrated. We may overeat, stuffing our frustrations by filling our emptiness with food. We try to satisfy our inner being by compensating our bodies. It doesn't work. The cry from within only grows louder. HALP!

Even with this cry growing louder, we may deny the cry, covering it up so we don't have to face what it asks of us. We may be afraid that if we share our feelings someone else will judge us negatively. Fearing the criticism of others, we learn to be critical of ourselves. And as we judge ourselves critically, we judge others in the same way. We look for what lacks instead of what gives life. We look for people who are as confused as we are, so that we won't feel alone. We remain alone with our emptiness and feeling unlovable.

Then we talk about it, and it gets worse. Our critical voices give us no peace. We remain alone in emptiness, because we lack love. After all, love is what we are really searching for. Giving it, receiving it, filling our souls with it, we find our way to bliss.

As long as we walk other people's paths, we're not on our own path. Our own path is the only path that will open our hearts and allow us to listen for its love song. You have within you the freedom to give and receive love every minute of every day. Your love is in your heart. How can you find that inner rhythm? Ask your heart, then listen for its song.

The Cry for Help is a Cry for Love

Our inner voice is crying out to us, crying for a wisdom that is bigger than us. It's calling for a way out of the discomfort. Why do we resist this? For some reason we fear the knowledge that could take us out of the vicious cycle of despair and denial. We resist the knowledge, instead eating, drinking, smoking, staying addicted to our old habits. The old habits seemed to give us comfort, but in the end they weren't the answer to what we really want or what we really need. We listen to everyone's opinion but our own. We just got stuck. Now the cry from inside says: "Make a new start. Listen to your own heart."

When I need to really think things through, I put a small tablet and a pen in my pocket, focus on my heart, and sincerely ask,

> *How can I solve this problem?*
> *How can I do this better?*

Then rain, sunshine, or snow, out the door I go. Every kind of weather stimulates our senses. I detach from whatever problem it is and surrender it. I tell myself,

> *Oh, dear God, I give this problem to you. It is bigger than me.*

As I walk, I ask for help, love, and an answer. Then I let it go. I look around me, noticing the trees, the weather, ducks or cats or children or cars I pass by. I breathe deeply, letting go of the stress I hold in my solar plexus. So I breath deeply in and deeply and slowly out. After only a few minutes, my body begins to respond to my breathing. I feel more calm. My racing thoughts slow down. I am aware of my breath and observe everything around me.

Then the feelings come, and I let them. If I'm sad, I cry. If I'm angry, I write in my notebook that I'm angry, or if I'm alone I say it out loud. As Elisabeth Kübler-Ross writes in her books about grief, we usually go through several stages of feelings before coming to serenity. First we are angry, then sad, then disappointed, then confused, then angry again. Believe it or not, this is a normal and natural process. Feeling and acknowledging the range of emotions flushes them out. When I feel hurt by others, my whole body feels the pain. Now with the rhythm of my arms swinging back and forth and my legs moving me forward, I air out what blocks me inside. When this is clear, I am ready to hear the answers that higher wisdom intends for me.

My little tablet comes out of my pocket as I find a place to sit down. Usually it takes only 20 minutes before I'm really to think differently about a problem or a challenge. I sometimes don't want to go on this walk, but I do it anyway because I always know I'll change for the better. It may take having a good cry in the forest or in my car on the way home. Oh, that is such a good release. Then I know God is answering. The release comes and new insights come. This is better by far than eating something or taking some medicine or even starting to think negative again, because when we start thinking negative, you know the spiral starts....downward. Yesterday I noticed a million sunflowers growing in a field all looking to the sun. Need I say more?

I get energy from this walking and noticing and breathing. Afterward I'm glad I went, and that's all that matters. Do it when you want. Nothing is a must! Do have the courage to try.

Now we start from the inside and go out to the path of enlightenment, turning on the light that shines from within. Now we are ready—ready to go on.

What Are You Seeking?

We are ever seeking the good feelings of life—peacefulness, serenity, happiness, warmth and comfort. A key to keeping your ideal weight is being in touch with what you really seek. To do this, you must allow yourself to feel your emotions. Feel them, for they are trying to send you a message of truth to your Soul, your Spirit, a message about the self you desire to be. To find these feelings, we peel away those layers of judgment and criticism to find the loving, all-accepting self within. The name we give to that pure self is the self of higher consciousness. We could say we're looking for a new inner self.

It makes sense. Our self ignites sparks of feelings. Our experiences and memories ignite sparks of feelings. Our all-knowing, wise hearts send us sparks of feelings. You wake up and see the sun shining and a smile comes to your face. You see a friend and she tells you some good news. You feel a rush of joy. Then the telephone rings and you learn a friend is sick. Your joy gives way to sadness and worry for your friend, thoughts of what you can do to help your friend, hope that she'll be well again soon, and gratitude for your own health. You may feel overwhelmed and fearful about the news. What will the future bring for her? What will the future bring for you?

These sparks of feelings merge in us creating new ideas and new convictions. These sparks can also lead us to make new decisions toward a path of love and change.

Find the Center of Your Spirit

Even as we look outside ourselves for inspiration, we also know that our deepest, most meaningful inspiration comes from within. Each of us divinely inspired in a unique way, we all have the same goal: joy, peace and love.

Accumulated experience and learning over many years contribute to a wealth of understanding of the complicated problems, solutions, and awakenings that can occur every day. I am grateful every day that this experience and insight can create a path to the higher self. Like stepping stones, experiences and insights let me step lightly to my destiny, with love in my heart and an intention to give back all that I've learned.

I also know it is important to acknowledge my deep respect and give credit to all the people who pass through my life on the way to their desires. They deserve the highest adoration for touching my heart and I theirs.

When I see that people are being encouraged because of what I share with them, I am grateful to the higher power I consider always evident in my life, the lives of others, and the universe. I believe I am transferring grace and power to others from a source higher than myself. They are also sharing their precious spirit with me.

Trust Your Process

When problems surface, I sometimes respond in just the same way as those who come to me for help. Sometimes I wait until I am in pain before I ask for spiritual help and guidance, yet I know that when I do ask for solutions, guidance and direction, an answer always comes to me. The answer is not always a simple one. I'll get an insight, not necessarily a voice, but a *knowing*. It will dawn on me to stop focusing on the problem I am faced with and instead ask my higher self for the solution. Someone will tell me, "Mary, listen to your inner self. It knows everything."

Now where do these answers come from? How do we always seem to get the right answer at the right time? I believe there is a force or source that is larger than myself, and this force is behind a purpose or destiny toward which I am traveling through life. I have also noticed that when I trust the process of growth, allowing it to unfold in a natural way, a feeling of calmness or oneness with the universe comes over me.

Give yourself a space to just listen to the messages that rise up out of the silence. This is an example of trusting your life. You can't force inner awareness. You can't schedule it the way you can schedule an appointment. Your inner life works not on time but on desire. Trusting that your desire will lead you to the right place at the right time is the beginning of finding grace.

Trusting yourself connects you to the realm of spirit. When I trust my own soul process, I feel as if I can trust the very essence from which all my thoughts and dreams are coming. When I have this calm understanding that I can trust the universe for literally everything, my body relaxes. I can trust that I will be given all the love I need, all the security and all the knowledge to pursue my own destiny, and my mind becomes clear to receive what I need. When I worry that I won't get what I need or create a fear or illusion of failure, I shut down inside. I stand in the way of my own success, the success that I will be given if I am ready and willing to receive it.

A Higher Purpose, a True Destiny

I wasn't destined to be overweight. Are you? I use myself as an example here because for years, perhaps like some of you, I did not know I could be really in control of becoming the person I wanted to be. I had the idea that I was destined to be overweight. I thought that was just the way my life was supposed to be. I tried every new diet book that came out, all the quick fixes from magazines, ate only grapefruit then switched to cucumbers, fasted, and counted calories and grams. And I was still fat.

I finally found out that I could place my thought and desire into the universe, turn it over to my higher power, and be willing to *allow* it to happen rather than rely on other people to tell me how to lose weight. There is a big difference between demanding a result without *fully committing* yourself and being *willing* to do whatever is necessary to get to that result. In that fullness of willingness that goes through every fiber of your being—your head, heart, stomach, hands, eyes, soul—you will feel a willingness to *allow* your intentions to become realities. The difference is that your whole being supports your dreams. You find faith and trust in yourself, maybe for the first time in your life.

A man named Peter came to my seminar to lose weight. He was a computer programmer and hated his work. He worked day and night perfecting computer programs while his body grew bigger and bigger. Food was the only thing that helped him get through the work. One day in the seminar we talked about creativity and doing work we love. "Doing creative work is like being in love. Peter," I asked. "What would you love to do? Do you have a hobby?"

"I like photography," he replied, smiling. His face lit up when he mentioned it.

Everyone in the group said, "Peter, you have to pursue that!" That was the last day of the seminar, but here the story gets better.

About a year later, I was in the central train station buying a train ticket, and here came a man with cameras hanging around his neck, running to catch a train. It was Peter! Astounded, I yelled after him: "Peter, is that you?!"

As he ran by, he smiled and yelled, "Hoi, Mary! I lost 27 kilos! Bye...I'm going to a photo shoot!"

I called after him, "No more computers?"

He yelled back, "Never!"

Peter had found his creativity and the heart of his wellbeing. Sometimes while I am walking in the mountains looking at nature's beauty, hearing rushing streams and feeling the Earth under my feet, all of my senses make me aware that everything around me is operating in perfect harmony. It's all humming along with some kind of force or source that is larger than life as we understand it. And even more, while in the beauty of nature, I notice that nature knows how to create magnificent miracles. When I notice an army of ants, for example, all on a mission, with a purpose, all in line carrying supplies to a special place to function and survive, I can't help but wonder if each of us also has a purpose and mission.

I believe my purpose is to carry a message to delight to others that can enable them to transcend toward greater joy. This purpose puts my desires in perfect harmony with everyone and everything else. We transcend together. Transformations come in relationship to all people we come in contact with and the world. When we change our body from what we don't want to what we do want, we transform. You will not be the same person you were before you read this book. You are not the same today as you were yesterday, or even the same as you were an hour ago.

You are changing, as we all are. In this amazing process, you are not alone. As soon as I am conscious of you, and you are conscious of me, we are together in spirit. I am with you in the process of evolving toward a higher purpose and a higher self.

This notion of a higher source or power is not the kind of thing you can measure or relate to facts. None of us really knows exactly what this spiritual power is, but all of us, in our own way, know that it exists.

For thousands of years philosophers have put labels on it, formed churches and temples, and spent lifetimes trying to capture its essence. Millions of people in various religions have developed their own ways to capture the spiritual.

There seems to be comfort at all levels of understanding that we are not alone in this world but rather bonded together by the belief in a power larger than ourselves. Our bonding can offer comfort in dark times and lift us back to a light, joyful state, when we willingly allow it to come into our hearts.

When we fall into the illusion of being out of control or powerless to master our own destinies, there seems to be a guiding influence that gives us knowledge of the right path to take in order to restore our balance and harmony. Some people call it an awakening or a vision.

I am not trying to promote any specific religion or way of worship, because for some this larger-than-life experience can be as simple as a hunch or an intuition, a thought or idea or a special attentiveness to everyday life. It doesn't matter where it comes from, as long as it gives us the power to go forward, creating a destiny that contributes meaning to our happiness and fulfillment—our peace.

Losing extra weight and becoming healthier can create a balance of energy and movement as we breathe the fullness of life into our bodies with a lighthearted energy. It enables us to respond to ideas and thoughts from the universe and to ask for help. We learn to open up to the harmony with all living beings that can lead us to our destiny, for we are part of that harmony.

We can *ask* for courage, faith and motivation, believing we can rely on our higher source. We can open the door to the knowledge of our own resources from within ourselves, or the universe, allowing us to accept ourselves as harmonious with the very nature of life. Or, we can wonder, worry, obsess and eat a lot of extra food. We are the choice makers.

Faith is the Seed of Personal Power

The importance of acknowledging a higher power is not to label it or debate it but rather to consider it as the prime cause for your destiny to succeed. When you believe this, you are not alone. If there are any such things as miracles, they are produced through the state of mind known as faith.

Here's an example of the power of faith demonstrated by a man known throughout the world, Mahatma Gandhi. In this man the world had one of the most outstanding examples known to civilization of the possibilities of faith. Gandhi had a tremendous amount of power, despite the fact that he used none of the conventional tools of power, such as money, soldiers, and guns. So how did Gandhi come by the power that inspired so many people over so many years to follow his guidance?

Gandhi created a following out of his own understanding of faith and through his ability to transplant that faith into the minds of many millions of people. Gandhi influenced all these people to move in peaceful unison as a *single mind*. What other force on Earth, except faith, could do as much? Faith can transform desire into a physical event, as Gandhi proved and as you prove every day that you stick to your own personal destiny, whatever that may be. That transformation comes right down to your faith in yourself, your purpose, and your trust in a higher power as you understand it.

When faith is blended with thought, the unconscious mind instantly picks up the vibration. You can create faith in yourself with your affirmations and repeating your belief statements. Repeating your beliefs in silence will plant a seed of faith that will blossom and grow. You will be stronger. You will be more serene. When you dominate your mind with your intentions, you give your subconscious the messages and desires. By taking action every day, faith in yourself grows stronger and stronger. You begin to feel more harmonious and more motivated, with a positive outlook on everything that you seek to find, everything that you seek to accomplish.

Each day, as you continue toward your desire to lose weight, be willing to let go of your old habits about your overweight condition, as if you are shedding an old skin. You are transcending your past seasons from your wall of protection and emptiness to a new awareness of all that you are. Each day as you have more faith and trust in yourself and your decision to reach your ideal weight, allow yourself to evolve into the healthy, thinner person you choose to be. Remember, you already have all the resources you need within yourself.

Becoming Intimate with Our Inner Selves

We think of being intimate with other people, but we usually don't think of being intimate with ourselves. We think that because we live with ourselves every day, we know everything there is to know. But we are intimate mysteries, full of surprising emotions, ideas and possibilities, if only we'll let ourselves see them.

The sheer beauty of Switzerland's nature first caused me to think about a wisdom greater than myself. I was visiting Switzerland, and the first sight of these towering mountains from a distance were so magnificent. Up close, I found delicate flowers blooming through the snow. What a miracle this seemed, strength and tenderness hand in hand in the landscape. My visit ended, and I went back to Houston, Texas, where I was trying to raise three boys on my own and start a career. It was a time in America when women wanted it all. I was caught up in this cultural idea that I had to be Superwoman. Houston was a huge city of 2.5 million people often terribly hot. I returned to this barren place after being in Switzerland, and a little voice inside me said, "Stop this and get out." I was crying out for help to my higher self or God. I didn't even know what to call it then. I remember driving around the hospital where I worked saying to myself, "I don't know what the future holds, but please, Dear God, not this for the rest of my life."

In the following years after the vision of the red cable car I threw myself into the unknown. That risk brought me to Switzerland, to letting go of my extra weight, to leaving behind the weight on my heart, to writing *Für Immer Schlank*, to meeting ten thousand people in my weight reduction courses, and to the book you are reading right now. We never know where the unknown will lead, but it always begins with being aware of feelings and having courage to honor the guiding power within.

Being aware from this stillpoint inside myself, I could observe my own feelings. Instead of being afraid, I could begin to ask, "What's the message? What is my soul trying to tell me?" My inner voice could begin to speak without fear that I would silence it: "That thought isn't acceptable. That's not possible!" Instead, I could begin to hear and just let the messages come without judgement. When the voice became clear, I could no longer resist the change I knew in my heart I had to make. I believe that had I stayed in Houston, I would have died.

Intimacy with our feelings, especially difficult feelings, is one of the most difficult transformations we can make in our lives. Relaxation, meditation, and observing feelings isn't a way to escape from these feelings but a way to merge with them and move through them. It's like driving on the autobahn through the fog. Sometimes you can only see one meter in front of you. Then the fog clears for a moment, and you breathe a sigh of relief. In the next minute, the fog closes in and you're back to a slow pace, creeping through wondering when you'll have a clear vision again. You may be afraid to drive with such limited vision. But you move through it. It's a process.

Facing difficult emotions, especially fear, is like driving through the fog. Perhaps you look at brave people and think, "They're brave because they have no fear. They're not like me." The truth is that they are intimate with fear. They take a deep breath and begin driving through the fog the best they can, knowing that they will reach a time when the fog will lift and they will find themselves on the path of their own inner heart. Being intimate with fear is a sign of honesty with ourselves. Willing to hear the message it has for us, we also open the way to hear the other messages of our heart: the messages of love.

I'm reminded of a story I heard from American philosopher Wayne Dyer. In the late 1800s, people blazed trails across the American West, searching for new opportunities and new horizons. Stagecoaches, pulled by teams of horses, carried mail and people over these new trails. The people who traveled in those stagecoaches didn't know what they'd find at the end of the trail, because they had never been there before. They were fueled by the anticipation and hope for a new future, full of dreams and fears.

Leaning out the window of the stagecoach, the passengers would see the backs of four horses who were running as hard as they could, their tails floating behind them, pulling the stagecoach on the bumpy path. The horses, out in front, pulled them into the unknown. Those horses are like our senses and feelings, running ahead of our conscious minds. The horses sensed danger before anyone in the coach, and they also were the first to sense lifegiving water along the way. The driver, with the reins in hand, is like our conscious mind, trying to steer the wild energy of our feelings. Our emotions, like the horses, would take us off the path if the driver let them. The driver, with a tug on one rein or the other, keeps the momentum moving in the right direction toward the destination. Inside the coach, which is like our bodies, is the passenger, which is our Self. The Self set the course at the beginning of the trip, and now she trusts the conscious mind and emotions to take the body where it needs to go. She directs them silently with her intention and her desire for the destination. As the coach rocks back and forth through unknown territory, the passenger thinks of the new place that awaits her at the end of the road. She smiles to herself, and silently urges the driver and horses on to bring her there safely.

Each of is on this path into new territory. How can I really tell you how to find your own path? How to harness your desires and emotions to take you there? How can I tell you how to direct your forward move-ment into the future that you want? Our basic instinct tells us to run away from the unknown. But running from the unknown is the same as running from the best possibilities that await us. What treasure is hidden in your future? You'll never know unless you dare to look. You can take the first step.

Pause for a moment. Take a deep breath and let the stress of the day and the fear of the future drop away like an old coat. Feel the lightness and strength of your emotions, your conscious mind, your Self. Feel them reach together toward the destination that is coming into view. Do you see it? Do you feel it? The warmth isn't only from without but also from within. Love is on the horizon, coming close. Spirit is everywhere, giving your dream wings. You are entering the realm of your Soul. Here is where you find peace. This unknown territory no longer seems strange, because this is your future, and it's filled with love.

Remember Your Divine Purpose

Why are you here today, reading this book in this very moment? You're here because you're a seeker. You are here hoping to find something you don't have. But what are you seeking? A secret to weight loss? Some special knowledge that will help you find that sense of physical balance you've probably been seeking for a long time? Maybe you're here seeking support from the group so you can put into practice what you may already have a hunch is the right way to live so you can reach your ideal weight.

We seek because we have needs. We have desires. I need. I want. I hunger. We have longings in our bodies. We have longings in our minds and souls. We want more...but more of what? We may want more food, but we've learned that doesn't really satisfy the hunger. Have you ever stood in front of the refrigerator with the door open asking, "What do I want?" The refrigerator is full, but you sense that what you want isn't in there. It's not outside you. It's you.

Is it possible we really want more of *ourselves?*

Food is an amazing substance. We can't live without it, and some of us have had experiences that show we don't know how to live *with* it! After a full meal, we can feel wholly satisfied...or depressingly empty. What's going on? Is it the food? Or is it our relationship to food? Is it what the food does to us or is it the intention we bring to the food?

Let's open the field wider, and I'll ask again: what are we all seeking? What do you want that's related to your body besides reaching your ideal weight? What do you want that's related to your mind? Your spirit? What do you want that's related to other people? What do you really want for you? How do these things we want make us feel? Do they give us pain or pleasure?

Pleasure, of course. If we think about it in this light, most of our daily life is filled with activities that in one way or another are about seeking pleasure. We want to feel good, and that means feeling good about ourselves. We want to be able to like ourselves, the way we look, the way we act, the way others regard us. We want to feel comfort. We want to feel secure. We also want to be able to help others feel secure. We want to be able to give *and* receive the most intimate, trusting feelings and live a life that reflects those feelings. We want to be loved.

When we're living and acting out of these pleasurable feelings, we can become satisfied. We can become whole. We begin to realize our potential in ways that we never imagined before. We begin to tap into the field of infinite possibilities, where barriers come down and we begin to become the person we have always wanted to be. We find our Ideal weight, better health, more loving relationships, more creativity...so much is waiting in that place. It is there that we can feel and act *fully* human, fully giving, fully loving and being loved.

In our culture, however, seeking pleasure is usually seen as a self-centered activity that is at the expense of other people, and keeps us psychologically and emotionally in an immature state. Indeed, if we seek pleasure *only* for the purpose of avoiding pain, then pleasure can become a substance of addiction. If we expect that buying something new is going to solve our relationship problems, we could be unaware of what we really want. If we think that a few cookies will make us feel better, it could be a childhood memory.

So we are going to understand that seeking pleasure is the beginning of a path that brings us into greater connection with ourselves, with other people, and with the Divine inside us. It's a first step toward opening our hearts to possibilities that we can't reach any other way. We can use it as a tool for motivation and it can help us face—not avoid—the difficulties that everyone faces from time to time.

Because life isn't always pleasurable. We all know that. Do we all like ourselves 100% of the time? Do we always do what's best for ourselves and others? Are our relationships always loving? Do we always follow through on our loving commitments to ourselves? Life isn't always so simple. Stress bears down from so many different directions. We may lose a job. We may have to move. Someone we love leaves or is taken from us. We do our best, but we feel misunderstood, even guilty or not good enough. We do our best, but sometimes we feel we haven't done enough.

The disappointment, that feeling in our gut that says things have gone badly, is a horrible feeling. And that can trigger, for many of us, a trigger to compensate that feeling with something that is pleasurable. When we feel bad inside, it has been a typical response to look outside of ourselves for the answer. For many of us, that compensating pleasure has been food—but that's not what we really needed.

The food may make us feel better in the short-term, but as weight is gained and the clothes get tighter, it only adds to our pain instead of supporting our search for pleasure. What's the answer? A diet? You just have to look at all the diets that are available to know that they're not working. Typical diets create a sense of deprivation that feeds pain, not pleasure. Your ideal weight can integrate with your daily life in a way that you can maintain forever. Like the short-term pleasure you get from eating that chocolate in a stressful moment, a diet is a short-term solution that rarely lasts. The weight comes back, and you face the same dilemma as always. This is the yo-yo diet syndrome. If you've experienced the yo-yo, you're not alone.

So how can you change this cycle? Essentially, ideal weight helps you to unlearn the old habits and ways of thinking that kept you trapped and help you find the wholeness, acceptance within yourself, and a practical structure for living that supports your ideal weight. Instead of seeking *pleasure in food*, you can balance that with seeking your heart's desire in all of life.

This isn't simple compensation, trading one sensory pleasure for another. The pleasures you will find now are in the realms of body, mind and spirit. To discover them, you will explore your own desires and intentions in ways that expand how you view yourself and the world. You'll learn to see yourself as a seeker of love, a person capable of infinite creativity, fully loving and lovable.

Set Yourself Free

In the Bible it says, "Life happens as you believe." It says that if you have the faith of a mustard seed, you can move mountains. As a child, I wondered what all that meant. Move a mountain? I lived in Minnesota where there aren't any mountains, but even I had seen pictures of the Alps, and I knew you couldn't just pick up a mountain and move it.

So what did it mean? I even wore a mustard seed around my neck, just in case it worked. Over the years I struggled to untangle this beautiful metaphor. After all, for thousands of years people all over the world have lived their lives by this simple statement, or at least tried to. So I wondered...what if I were the mustard seed? What if I simply let myself grow and bloom and somehow that force was great enough to move mountains? Maybe the force of one living, energetic being is strong enough to change the reality of even the biggest thing I can imagine.

I'm sure you've seen someone standing defiantly with his arms crossed, a little frown on his face, saying, "I'll believe it when I see it." Think about this person's stance. He has already decided that this event will probably not happen. He's already decided that it's just not possible. His arms are closed tight, protecting his body against the knowledge that he might have it backwards: that he indeed won't see until he allows the possibility.

When we start each day armed with doubt and skepticism, we show ourselves and the world that we are not really ready to accept the bounty that could be ours. The result? We don't get what we ask for.

You may feel this way about your attempts at reducing your weight. If you've lost and gained weight over and over again, it's easy to have a skeptical attitude. I can understand why you might feel this way, but I want to tell you, right now, that if you believe you will eventually fail, then indeed you will give up. But what if you woke up every morning and said

"I'll see it when I believe it."

What you believe creates your reality. Simply becoming aware of new thoughts begins the process of their manifestation in your life.

Open your heart to your positive possibilities while you let go of what restrains you. Right at this moment, you may be thinking about your own possibilities and capabilities. You may be thinking, "I can do this," or, "I can't do this." Remember, a belief is an idea that has the force of certainty behind it. A belief feels true to you.

Your beliefs either align your inner state with your outer actions or create conflict. If you say, "I can do that," your belief in that possibility causes your brain to deliver a direct command to your nervous system that sets your physical being in motion to support that inner state. If, on the other hand, you have a belief that goes against an outside intention, you will create a state of conflict in yourself that will feel like a battle being waged inside you. This is the typical state that diets create.

You have decided to follow the learning in this book to reach the vision of your ideal weight. You are taking specific, physical steps to make that happen. But if, inside, you actually believe that you won't succeed, you will find yourself struggling to maintain your vision. It will fade in and out of your mind's eye in response to your doubt. Your doubt is like interference on a radio transmitter. The signal of your success can't come in clearly if your mind and heart are filled with the static of doubt and disbelief!

When you really begin to allow the success of your steps, you create an inner state which allows it to become true on the outside. Whether you say you can or say you can't—you are right. "I can't do it" really means "I will not allow it." "I can do it" means "I'm creating the certainty of my desires." Whatever you choose to believe is true. Your belief controls your reality.

Belief gives us energy to help us act in certain ways. We can believe in success or simply in the possibility of success. If you believe in success, you will be empowered to achieve it. If you believe in failure, the messages you give yourself will lead you to experience that instead. If you believe that something is possible in your life, you open a door through which it can enter. If you believe that you can't change, you certainly won't.

Just as you can propel yourself forward into a bright future with positive thoughts, you can keep yourself stuck in the muck of limiting beliefs. You make the choice. You can choose beliefs that limit or beliefs that support your intentions and desires.

For as many reasons as you want to be thinner, you have reasons why you aren't thinner now. Read the following statements and ask yourself if you've heard them anywhere before. Maybe you've even said some of them yourself (I know I have):

"I can't lose weight because I'm just like my mother/father, and she/he was/is overweight."

"I can't lose weight because I have to cook for my children and eat with them to be a good example."

"I can't lose weight because I have to give dinner parties, and it wouldn't be polite not to eat!"

"I can't lose weight because I have big bones."

"I can't lose weight because all the people in my family are big."

"I can't lose weight because I'm lazy."

"I can't lose weight because I don't have enough willpower."

"Every time I lose weight, I gain it back."

"I can't lose weight because I eat too much."

"I can't lose weight because I just can't control myself around food."

"I can't lose weight because I can't say 'no' at a restaurant or at a party."

"I can't lose weight because I think too much about eating."

"I can't lose weight because I eat when I'm bored/angry/happy/sad."

"I can't lose weight because I just can't throw food on my plate (or anyone else's plates) away."

"I can't lose weight because I'm too busy! I just don't have time to watch what I eat or exercise."

"I can't lose weight because if I just look at food, it goes to my thighs."

"I eat the same amount as other people. I can't lose weight because I have a slow metabolism."

"I can't lose weight because I was born with fat genes. This is just the way I am."

Do any of these sound familiar? These statements can seem like the truth. But these limiting beliefs—and everything you just read is only a belief that someone has chosen to adopt—are just some of the things we say to convince ourselves that we have to be overweight and that we have no choice about it.

One woman in my seminars successfully followed her plan to stay in the new shoes for three weeks. I counsel my seminar-goers not to weigh themselves too often and, instead, to concentrate on how they are feeling. I say this to you, too!

This woman weighed herself every day, and the scale did show that she was consistently losing weight. But, as the scale read fewer and fewer kilos, she became more and more anxious. She couldn't believe that she was actually losing weight, so she convinced herself that her scale was broken. She went out and bought a new scale, but the new scale read the same as the old 'broken' one.

She came to me, frustrated, and told me this story. I asked her why it was so hard for her to believe that she was losing weight.

"Because I can't lose weight! It always comes back!" She was near tears. Oh, dear friend…we talked some more, and she discovered that she hadn't been weighing herself to measure her success—she was weighing herself to see if she was failing!

For the next week, she concentrated on positive beliefs. She made a conscious decision to let go of her doubts. She came the next week and said she had gotten rid of both scales. She didn't want to concentrate on kilos anymore, because she associated that with the unsuccessful results of all her previous attempts to shed the extra weight.

Where Do Beliefs Come From?

Every day we wake up with the set of thoughts that defines what we feel is possible in our lives. These are beliefs. So why do some people have beliefs that push them toward success while others have beliefs that lead them toward failure? Why do some people believe that everything is possible while others believe that we are born to suffer, powerless and unable to change our destiny?

Most beliefs come out of our history. We adopted them from the people we loved. We wanted their love and acceptance, so we modeled ourselves after them, acting in a way that reflected what they valued. In this way, their beliefs became our beliefs. This made us feel connected and loved.

My parents believed that being big and strong was a good thing. To be big and strong, they believed, you should eat a lot. So, I believed it too, and I ate a lot, even though it was more than I needed and made me overweight. I believed them because they were my parents. I loved them and wanted their approval. When I ate, they praised me, and I knew they were happy with me.

As an adult, long after I had left home and established my own family, I was still eating in this same way. The same big portions that left me feeling stuffed, the same feeling that somehow I was being good by eating all this food…but my parents were no longer around to nod to each other and smile on me. The reason for the belief was gone, but the behavior stuck!

Beliefs we learned as children can feel so deep that we can't even remember a time when we didn't have the belief. When our entire personal history is framed by a belief, it's hard to see it separate from ourselves. It feels like a foundation block of our sense of self, even if it's one that harms our health and wellbeing. It feels like we were born with these forceful beliefs in the same way we were born with fingers and toes.

"Good girls and boys eat everything on their plates."

"A meal isn't healthy unless it has big portions of every food group."

"Eat it all up."

"Having a cookie will make you feel better."

"Eating a big family meal together shows how much we love each other."

"If you eat all the food on your plate, then you deserve to have dessert."

Though it may feel like our beliefs are an inextricable part of our being, we were not born with them. We learned them, and that means that we can unlearn them, let them go, and replace them with ideas that suit us better in this phase of life. We can begin now.

Every Belief Is Based In A Positive Intention

Every belief that we learn has a positive intention. Our parents' positive intention was to make us behave, show us they loved us, and to give us what they thought were good eating habits.

There's no point in blaming anyone. Our parents and teachers taught us from the beliefs that they learned from their parents and teachers. We all do the best we can in the moment. Just as you are striving to do the best you can, realize that they, in their own ways, were too.

On the strength of that early training, old beliefs about eating will almost always continue until we make a conscious decision to change. Until that time, we continue to act out ideas that were planted years ago, even though they no longer serve any useful purpose in our lives. Let me tell you a story, from my own experience, about a limiting belief that kept me overweight for years.

My mother makes delicious cookies and cakes. I can't count the number of times I came into the house and was guided to the kitchen by the smells of cookies and cakes baking. There she would be, busily baking something to carry down the street to someone who was ill, sad, or lonely. She baked for church, school, and community gatherings. She seemed to always be in the kitchen, with warm aromas floating through the house.

I can't remember a time when there were no cookies in the house. They were always stored in odd-shaped tins of a dozen different sizes, ready to be offered should someone drop in for coffee. For years and years, conversations were centered around the kitchen table with coffee and plates of cookies.

Needless to say, I consumed hundreds, or maybe thousands, of cookies over the years while puzzling out problems and emotional issues with absolutely no notion that these delights were contributing to my ever-growing weight problem.

As a wife and mother, I too began baking cookies, and I really believed they were helping to soothe my pain! I didn't think of eating as a distraction. It was the path to a solution! My belief about the power of a cookie to heal my pain turned into a habit that, while giving me momentary gratification, left me with bigger problems—too much weight and too little self-esteem!

I've come to realize, through the experience of giving seminars, that many, many people have a similar belief that problems are soothed—or even solved—by eating.

I no longer believe that food solves problems, and so when I find myself in the middle of a stressful situation, I don't automatically think about reaching for a cookie, like I used to. When I believed that food would fix things, the first (and sometimes only) response to stress was how I could get my hands on a sweet, quick fix.

But remember that food is just food. It doesn't have any special power—*you* have the power.

Love People More than Food

Mother's Day and Easter are just two of the times during the year that many people resign themselves to overeating. Instead of being in control, most people are frantically doing 'damage control.' How many of us have heard,

"Just have one. It won't hurt you to have just one."

"I worked so hard on this dish! If you don't try it, you'll hurt my feelings."

"Oh, come on…you can diet with the rest of us *after* the holiday"

This kind of social pressure is common during holidays as well as at other times during the year. While your host, hostess and fellow party-goers have good intentions (they just want you to enjoy the holiday), they are also sending another message: "If you don't eat along with the rest of us, you won't have a good time."

Do you believe that? Do you go to parties just for the food? What about the camaraderie of family and friends? What about the stories that you will share together? Think about the memories that you are making. Do you want to remember the buffet table or do you want to remember the warmth and laughter of friends. Every gathering can be a circle of spirit, if you choose to focus on the love that you all have to share.

You do have a choice. You can choose to say, "Thanks, I have enough. Tell me what's been going on in your life?" Think how you'll feel knowing that food is just food, and that the real life of the holiday is in your connection with other people and with your spiritual self.

Too much food is a diversion from life. When we give food the power of emotional healing, we are only diverting ourselves from our real task. We avoid dealing head on with our problems by sidestepping them, handing them over to a cookie or muffin or second helping that only buries our conflict under another layer of fat.

The Diet of Forgiveness

Loving is not always as easy as we hope. We fear being hurt. We fear opening ourselves up to someone who may not love us in return. Hasn't everyone been wounded in this way? I'm sure we have all paid a visit to Heartbreak Hotel once or twice. We've all experienced the disappointment of not getting something we longed for so much. We've all experienced the pain of friendships gone wrong. The pain, so excruciating, can sometimes feel like a kind of death. When it becomes too hard to bear we survive by denying the pain and just stuffing our feelings deep inside. Time wears away the trauma, and we harbor the resentment like smoldering coals in our hearts. The hurts never seems to go away.

And indeed the hurt will never go away as long as we hold it in our hearts. Now's the time to let go. I think we have suffered enough from memories left over from yesterday. They are just too heavy to carry. Do you know why I really think forgiving and being forgiven is important? So that we can mend our broken hearts. Earlier I said fear of loss is one of the greatest fears we have. Loss of what? Loss of love. Of all the broken hearts we have suffered through, it was always true that the suffering was because of a lack of love or loss of love.

The memory of loss of love is the very thing that makes us afraid to fall in love again, even with ourselves. So we resist the very most important ingredient in life, love. We even build a protection of fat around ourselves to protect ourselves from love and the impending loss of it. So here we are in resistance of what we desire more than anything. Are we crazy? Sometimes it feels like it.

What if we were to release all of the fear and the resistance against love? We could do it with forgiveness, starting with forgiving ourselves for being overweight. We could even forgive our mothers who encouraged us to eat and eat just to get dessert. What about those who betrayed us and the ones we betrayed? Couldn't we release the burden of resentment, reunite with ourselves and begin anew? It would be a decision, a big one.

By now you know that diets don't work, at least diets about eating. Even the word diet makes you cringe, but what if you could give new meaning to the word "diet," using it to mean a way of nurturing yourself instead of depriving yourself?

One day while walking in the mountains I was trying to help a friend who had a serious problem of overweight. That particular day she was very upset. I was looking for ideas to soothe her, and inside myself I was praying about this.

It was no coincidence that the night before I was reading a book I had bought a few years prior called *A Course In Miracles*. My friend was so resentful of her husband, stuck in the state of resentment. I began reading something to her that said: "Forgive seventy times seven." I wondered why it was that number and what it really meant. Seeking an answer I thought that maybe seventy times seven, which is 490, is how many forgiveness affirmations it would take to get serious about releasing the suppressed anger that she had carried for some 20 years. Saying an affirmation of forgiveness two or three times would never be enough to unlock the mind. But maybe seventy times seven would be enough.

An affirmation is a statement of certainty that you say over and over until you believe it is true. Affirmations can create the energy to jump out of a worn out state of mind that is holding you back from your happiness.

I asked Rabbi David Cooper how to make affirmations work. He said the spiritual meaning of seventy times seven is *completion*. Completion isn't the same as an ending—it's the beginning of a transformation. Yes, I wanted my friend and my clients also to have it. It means feeling complete, free of guilt and fear.

We all would be willing to do anything to feel complete, so we wouldn't have to worry any more. If you do something seventy times seven, it would show your intention was so clear that you really meant it. You would be reprogramming your thinking well enough for your Higher Power to hear that now you really mean you are ready. Then you would get all the energy you ever need to get your permanent result.

I realized that when forgiveness is complete, a flowing river of energy that is total love starts to release your resentment. You will feel so good so relieved that you would never again have to look for substitutes. I tried this exercise myself over and over before I give it to you, and it works. There is power in repetition.

Ritual: Release Resentments

Think of someone who you feel has wronged you. Think of a resentment from the past that continues to hold you back. Now, make an affirmation of forgiveness about that situation, for example:

I, Mary, forgive my father completely.

For one week, write or say one affirmation 70 times each day. You can do 35 in the morning and 35 in the evening. Here are other examples:

I am ready to give up all my anger and resentment against

_____.

I forgive myself for the wrong thinking that has kept me blocked.
I forgive myself for harming my body.
I forgive myself for accepting food when I wanted love.
I forgive myself completely.
I am ready to forgive those I used to blame for wronging me.

Try saying one forgiveness affirmation per week for four weeks. Choose affirmations that speak to your heart. After these four weeks, move into using affirmations to let go of what stands between you a completion. Choose one affirmation per week for four weeks. Here are examples:

I am willing to let go of all that stands between me and completion.
I am ready to give up all my anger and resentment now.
I am ready to relax and accept the energy of total love.
I can safely accept love for myself.
I can safely offer forgiveness to myself and others.
I am now releasing my fear of letting go of my weight.
I now give up self hate and self doubt.
I have the right to choose what I think because my mind is in every cell of my body.

After this series of affirmations, choose affirmations that complete your transformation to a fully loving being. Use any that speak to your heart, but remember that the power is in seventy times seven: say one affirmation 70 times each day for one week to feel its effect. Here are affirmations I use:

Today I choose to give love.

Today I choose to receive love.

Today I notice love in everyone I see.

I am certain that there is enough food and love for me.

My body has a natural tendency toward heal and beauty.

I like my body, and the more I like it, the more lovable it becomes.

Because I created my body, I can appreciate all the good things about it.

I have the right to say No without losing people's love

My body is an individual expression of me. I no longer have to work out family patterns in my body.

I love and accept myself completely.

I have the power to live at the weight I desire.

I love food because I know it cannot harm me.

Everything I eat is nourishing to my body and soul and never harms me.

I approve of myself for eating. I am a thin woman/man who can sit and eat slowly and stop before I am full.

I am gradually giving up food without worry or effort.

I enjoy being attractive.

I am ready to accept the joys of love without fear of guilt.

I stay more attractive with more and more wonderful energy.

I am willing to stop blaming myself and others for my problems.

It is safe for me to feel good.

There is no problem that I can't resolve with help from my higher self and asking help from Divine wisdom.

I am ready to relax and accept the energy that is total love.

I am now spiritually nourished.

I am now listening to my inner being, which has the answers I seek.

The Power of Imagination

Humans have the unique ability to see things not only as they are, but also as they can be. Through the power of imagination we can transform our reality to meet our dreams. I have never seen anything give a person as much energy as a vision that he or she is working to bring into reality. I have seen people give up sleep, food, and basic comforts for the sake of a project that they love. When people are in the grip of a vision, they are unstoppable. There is something very magical about a person dedicated to a purpose, something more precious than I can put into words.

The same energy that moved the Albert Einsteins and the Thomas Edisons to change the world is also within us. We all have that spark— that thought inside us which can draw us to our own excellence. All we have to do is be willing to listen to it and act upon it. Within you lie talents far greater than you have recognized and expressed. It is your imagination that can trigger those abilities. In other words, it is possible for you to create whatever you can imagine. When you imagine yourself thin, as if it has already become a reality, you are giving a signal to your subconscious mind that you are ready to make a change that sets those wheels in motion.

Through creative imagination, your mind has direct contact with your subconscious. The subconscious is the faculty through which hunches and inspirations are received, and it is through creative imagination that all new ideas come to you. It not only causes you to think about being thin, but you begin to realize that you are capable of becoming exactly who you want to be. If you squeeze an orange, you get orange juice.

Imagination is the workshop of the mind. If you think about it, all plans of losing weight have started in your mind. Creative imagination becomes sharper with use, just as any muscle or organ of the body develops through exercise.

With Love, We Have Enough

Some people seem to have a bottomless hunger for emotional and physical satisfaction. Do you know someone like this? They never seem to have enough of anything. Even when they are paying their bills, have plenty of food on the table, have a stable relationship, and everything else they could possibly need, they still ache with a dark emptiness.

They work obsessively to make sure that every detail is cared for. They lose sleep worrying that they forgot something. But even when their effort brings them bright rewards, they can't relax and enjoy them. They simply don't know what to do with good fortune and success. During the times that life is full of crisis, they understand their purpose. They scale the cliffs with tenacity and courage, but when they stand on the peak of success, they suddenly feel dizzy and fall back to the bottom. The fear that nothing is ever enough is a common attitude that keeps us from fully accepting that we can have abundance and success if we want them. This state of mind says only one thing: "you will never have enough. Whatever you have, you will lose."

This is a habit of suffering, and people who live with it live under a shadow. This old habit says that pain—not love—is the inevitable state of our existence. Spiritually empty, full of fear, this soul has no gateway into experiencing real love and serenity. With a conscious decision to open a space for love to enter, however, this habit of suffering can be dissolved. If you sense that you have a habit of suffering, open your heart with these affirmations:

> *I have the resources I need. They are inside me, and no one can take them away from me.*
> *The world is filled with opportunity.*
> *Nothing that is truly important to me can be taken from me.*
> *Today I have all that I need.*

I trust the universe to provide me with the resources and opportunities I need to be whole. I will creatively use those gifts with love and an open heart.

Learning from a Baby

Here's a story I tell in my seminars. I learned this from my own experience, and when I think of it, I'm filled with wonder.

Every child comes into the world in love. Each and every mother and father think their baby is a miracle of life, and of course that's the truth. The child is filled with love and warm milk from mother's breasts. From the very first day the child is made to feel as comfortable as possible and is nurtured and nourished. The child is loved and accepted no matter if she is crying or falling asleep in mother's arms. When discomforted by hunger or pain, mother and father rush to restore comfort as fast as possible. The child learns to feel secure.

Soon the baby begins to learn and develop. In just one year the baby begins to stand up, pulling herself up with the help of a chair or coffee table. What a miracle! At first her little legs wobble and shake, and the baby falls down crying in frustration. After a minute, the baby has recovered and relentlessly tries to stand up again. She falls down again, recovers, and tries again. Mother and father watch with excited anticipation for the first step.

The baby has no doubt. Rather, she displays over and over the will to stand up...full confidence renewed after every fall. This is learning combined with perseverance and sheer will. Each time the baby tries, her legs are strengthened a little more. She may fall, but she has made progress through the little bits of strength she builds with each attempt. Magically one day her legs are strong enough. The baby's long awaited moment comes, and joyfully the child takes her first step.

This is the beginning of a life of walking, running, stretching, and growing. The baby never looks back and says, "Well, now that I can walk, I'll go back to sitting and crawling." What a powerful metaphor for learning! As adults, sometimes our doubt overshadows our will to make our intentions into reality, and along the way we give up. We have somehow forgotten that perseverance, banishing the doubt, and never giving up holds the secret. A baby knows this secret instinctively. We used to know this instinctively, but somewhere along the way we forgot. No one told the baby that her wish to walk was not possible. But as adults, many people tell us that our wishes and dreams are impossible. With total freedom and support, the baby moved forward step by step. Nothing, neither worry nor lack of self confidence, stood in the baby's way.

How then did we forget this fearlessness and confidence in our capabilities? Just think what energy we could pull from inside ourselves if we were to remember the capabilities that come from within us and say, "I am going to achieve my ideal weight." Each day we remember that we as babies also had the desire to walk...and did it without hesitation. Somewhere along the way we lost faith in ourselves, faith in our desires, faith in our capable selves. I believe we can get that back, simply by remembering what is possible for such a little infant to accomplish.

A Fast of Negative Thinking

We've been talking about what we really want, what we really desire. Now imagine you could wake up tomorrow with a clean slate. No history to overcome. No habits to hurdle. No patterns to redraw. Imagine how innocent we would feel…like being reborn with the innocent mind and curiosity of a child. We wouldn't have fear or resistance against one way or another way. We wouldn't have the voices of other people whispering in our ears that this way is better than that way. We wouldn't be worried about whether we are on trend or behind the times. We wouldn't worry about whether we're the best or the fastest or the richest or the thinnest. We could just be ourselves, open to our possibilities and the path ahead of us.

Of course we can't completely erase our past—nor would we want to lose all the great memories that happened along the way!—but we can learn to cultivate a sense of openness and willingness to change. We can learn to let go of what stands in our way and embrace what supports us.

Indeed, in order to make room for something new to come into our lives, we first have to let go of what holds us back. To help a rose bush bloom, we first have to prune it. At first, the bush looks ugly, empty, thorny. We may wonder what good could come from cutting it back. Pruning the bush, though, has triggered the plant to send out new growth. Blooms like never before burst forth. It can be that way in our lives too.

You've made a decision to let go of parts of your lifestyle that stand in the way of your dreams. You've "pruned" your habits, and you may feel a little thorny right now. Changing a routine can be uncomfortable. Unlearning a habit that may be ingrained with years of repetition can feel absolutely unnatural. As you wait for the blossoming of your new habits, your daily routine may feel foreign to you. Hang on! Remember that just as the bare rose bush is busy inside creating the roses that will bloom weeks later, so too your body, mind and spirit are building a new Self that is more deeply connected to your higher self, a fusion of inner and outer purpose.

Letting go of your old ways makes way for the new. Be confident that you are emerging in due time. It may not be when you expect, but if you continue to water your new habits in healthy ways, letting go of the past will not seem like a sacrifice but will be a blessing. Have patience with yourself. Rome wasn't built in a day. Resentment comes back. Let them go again and again. Each time, it becomes easier.

Pruning = new growth!

Old Habits Can Still Call Like a Distant Echo

Sometimes we are tempted through habit and compulsive thinking to go back to the Old Shoes. Our senses connect us with the here and now and also take us down the pathways of memory. Sometimes a smell or a sound can take us straight back into another time and place and trigger behavior that we thought we had long ago left behind. It's easy to recognize when this is happening but much more difficult to actually stop the behavior. When we are reminded of the past, we relive those experiences again at the unconscious level. This is sometimes so subtle that it takes a conscious effort to get at the real cause of the behavior.

I woke one morning in May and had a fluttery feeling in my stomach. I had a hard time focusing my mind, and I felt anxious about something…but I wasn't sure what!

I lay quietly in my warm bed for a couple of minutes. I thought about other things—my desire to take a walk by the lake today, my work schedule for the day, my positive intentions to eat only what would help me stay at my ideal weight—and then I returned my attention to the anxiety that still ran like waves through my stomach.

This anxiety felt like…insecurity. I felt unprotected. But what was I feeling insecure about? Was it money? No. I had enough to pay my bills. Was I lonely? No. Was I afraid of the future? No, that wasn't it.

So what was it? I lay quietly for a few more minutes, thinking of other things.

Suddenly I remembered that in this exact month, two years ago, I had been feeling very insecure and with good reason. I was involved in a project that had nearly ruined me financially and had cost me a great deal in emotional and physical energy. It had been a cold and rainy spring, and I remember how I had gone over and over my situation while I took my spring clothes out of storage and packed the winter ones away.

Now, I lay in bed realizing that the previous night I had taken my spring clothes out and packed my winter ones away. And out with the spring clothes had come all those memories intact. The association between my feelings of insecurity and the act of unpacking my spring clothes was as direct as a telephone line.

I was thankful for awareness that emerged that morning. Without it, I would have been tempted to soothe my troubled emotions with the old habit of too much food. My stomach sure felt fluttery, and I could have easily mistaken this for real physical hunger or simply decided to drown the uncomfortable feeling with food.

Even though I realized consciously what feelings I was having again, it didn't mean they automatically went away. It required attention to recognize that an old memory was playing and then make a decision to come back to the present.

I have learned, through hard experience, that this process must be approached gently. It takes its own time. This is one reason why I never jump straight out of bed in the morning. If I hadn't allowed myself time to discover the truth behind those feelings, my head would have been in the refrigerator while my feet were still sliding into my slippers. Those quiet, thoughtful moments before I start the day are essential in letting the awareness of my emotions surface.

Please, please take this time whenever you need it! If you find yourself in the grip of a feeling, take just five minutes out of whatever you're doing to sit quietly with the feelings.

It can be a struggle just to allow yourself to take this time. There are always at least six other things you should be doing, and when you can't really explain what you're feeling, it can feel selfish to leave more definite needs to explore vague, as yet unnamed feelings.

But this is not selfishness. This is self-care. It is necessary if you are going to hear what your inner voice has to tell you. You don't have to explain it to anyone. You don't have to justify this time to anyone. You just have to believe that you deserve to take it when you need it.

Here are some other things that can help you through difficult moments:

- call a friend
- write about what's bothering you
- write a note of love and acceptance to yourself
- take a contemplative bath or shower
- walk by a lake or in another natural setting
- listen to some music that makes you feel good. Sing to it! Dance to it! What lifts your spirits? Do it now.
- if you're still in the grip of that pull to overeat, say to yourself, "This impulse will pass. This will pass."

Here are some other rituals I use to let go of what stands between me and serenity of mind.

Ritual: The Leaf on a Stream

Let go, let go, let go…What is holding you back? What is blocking your heart? Imagine it as a leaf on a stream, floating away gently. As you watch it go, sometimes it gets stuck on stones or gets wedged between sticks of wood, but as the current keeps on flowing finally the little leaf works its way. It floats freely down the river and flows out to the sea.

Ritual: Give it Away

Look in your closet. Have you been holding on to an old coat or jacket that you know you will never wear again? Put it in a bag and give it away to people who need it. Notice how you feel afterward. My experience is, if I really let an old pattern go, or an old memory, taking the time to throw an old coat away means it is really finished!

Fill the Gaps with Positive Thoughts

There's an old story about a sage who grappled centuries ago with the issue of negative thinking. He realized that if he allowed negative thoughts to control his life, he would never get to heaven. He acquired two stacks of pebbles, one dark and one light, which he placed outside his hut. Every time he had a negative thought, he'd take a pebble from the dark stack and place it in a pile. When he had a loving thought, he'd take a white pebble and place it in another pile.

In his youth, the dark pile was larger than the white pile. However, as he went on in life, the white pile began to grow high, eventually casting a shadow over the dark pile. By the time he was ready to depart this world at an advanced age, he had completely conquered his negative thinking.

Expecting yourself to think positively will help you succeed. If you expect yourself to let go of the extra weight, you will. You can feel your motivation or lack of it. Your Inner Self knows.

You are in the midst of a positive life change. You are making a commitment to your own health and wellbeing. You are becoming your own best friend, doing something just for you. You are doing something you've dreamed of doing for years.

Your attitude will have everything to do with how you handle this change in the coming weeks. Diet thinking creates a negative attitude, because it is an attitude of deprivation. A negative attitude will see everything as a problem, crisis, or failure. A positive attitude will see those same situations as an opportunity to learn.

Having a positive attitude doesn't mean that you have to be artificially happy all the time. People who smile through every life situation are often as out of touch with their true feelings as people who are depressed. The positive attitude I'm talking about is giving energy to what we can do with our lives—the positive potential in every one of us—instead of making excuses: "I haven't got time" or "I'm too old."

Optimism is an orientation of the heart, a way of approaching what life brings you that lets you turn every moment into an opportunity to grow and learn. An optimistic outlook sees the seeds of growth in situations others might call a failure. There is no failure. What you thought was failure was really giving up on yourself.

Reaching your ideal weight—like climbing a mountain—takes patience and time. Thinking about your desire and intention persistently creates small steps. No one would think of climbing The Matterhorn before taking on countless smaller hills to refine their technique and learn what it really takes to scale the difficult parts of the mountain.

So, are you sitting at the bottom of that mountain? A negative attitude at this second says, "I'm not capable. I'm going home and put on those old, comfortable shoes."

A positive thought might be, "What caused me to give up? Instead of trying to go the whole way at once, today I'll just take a few steps. It may take a little longer, but I won't fall, and I know I'll get there in safety. I'll do what I know I can do today."

Ritual: Watch Your Positive Thoughts Grow

Like the sage, you can watch your own positive thoughts grow. Get two cups and a pile of white beans and a pile of black beans. Keep them in your office, living room, kitchen, or wherever you spend time during the day. When you have a positive thought, put a white bean in the cup. A negative thought? Put a black bean in the other cup. See this clear picture of your thoughts, and work toward filling the cup with white. When one pile of beans is used up, pour them out and begin again. Watch how the white cup is filled more quickly than the black, when you direct your thoughts toward a loving path.

Live in Love

Being overweight begins not with our hand reaching for the food. It begins inside, when our heart is closed to our true potential. Maybe our heart is closed because we hurt inside—from childhood memories, from current relationships, from a loss we just can't get over, from somehow not feeling good enough. Whatever the reason, our heart is closed, and that turns life from the path of love to the path of emptiness and hunger of the soul.

When your heart is closed, the search for connection with Self and the Divine becomes an endless treadmill of looking outward for the praise and affirmation that we really need from inside. We may get on the consumer treadmill, buying the latest and best to impress others and convince ourselves that we're doing alright. "Look at all the great stuff I have—only the best for me..."

But do we have the best from ourselves? Do we honor ourselves in the best ways we can? Do we love ourselves enough to treat our bodies and minds with the same attention we lavish on other decisions in our lives? When we're lost to ourselves, we're lost to everyone. When we know ourselves, accept ourselves unconditionally, and make a commitment to know and grow our inner, Divine Self, the world opens up to us. Relationships can blossom. We can live fully in the world.

Now we make an about face—to look inward and pay attention to our souls, to find a new relationship with ourselves…a new intimacy with ourselves…and the original Divine Self. Working from the inside out, we understand our inward path more fully.

The food we eat nourishes us in the world. Food is a wonderful, sensual part of the gifts the earth offers. Who can resist the wonderful fragrance of fresh strawberry? The brilliant orange of a steaming yam? The bright green of perfectly cooked broccoli? These are experiences to be savored along the way. They are experiences to uplift our spirits and give us energy for the work ahead. Enjoy food. Enjoy life. Enjoy relationships. Find pleasure in the right measure from every area of experience. This is the root of satisfaction.

Let Go to Live

We let go of excess baggage at three levels: physically, mentally, and spiritually. We reach our ideal weight when we can release the need to suffer through our bodies. Instead of eating food we don't need, we nurture our bodies with healing walks in nature; soothing, scented baths; laughing deeply; and breathing in and out, in and out. We nurture our minds and spirits by being creative, loving, and giving.

Letting go is a process with has two dimensions. As we let go of what we don't need, we become more aware of what we do need. We hold on to what we value, and it becomes more precious as we realized it was with us all along even though it was out of sight. As we let go and our hearts open, new feelings emerge. We experience ourselves and the world anew. We spring into the unknown with courage.

We surrender ourselves to our desires, dreams, and wishes, trusting the uncertainty and knowing our infinite possibilities line the path. Our desires motivate our choice to let go, detach from the outcome, and surrender to the infinite possibilities we have not previously been aware of.

We are surrendering our attachment to substances and experiences. We observe ourselves, seeing our desires and path without judgement. We begin to see our special purpose in the world. Doubt and fear of being unlovable are banished as we give and receive love, living and being in love. There is no longer a place in our days for what isn't filled with love.

Here are two rituals to help you surrender to the path of love.

Ritual: Keeping Love Close

Who do you love? Who loves you? Get a tablet and write the answers down. Put the paper on your bathroom mirror, on your refrigerator, or keep it in your purse. Look at these messengers of love and allow memories of good times with them to fill you up.

Ritual: The Face of Love

Frame pictures of the people you love and keep them at your bedside. Keep small size pictures with you in your purse. Look at these faces to remind yourself of all the love that surrounds you.

The State of Our Imagination is the State of Our Life

I believe the essence of soul is creative, intuitive, joyful, inspired. All our desires and energy come from soul. Remember when your desire for your ideal weight was only a thought? That thought is transformed into action, and your body is transformed. The result you can see in the mirror, but the beginning was inside, in the loving, giving part of yourself. Your touchstone is your original vision of yourself at your ideal weight. If you should ever slip back into old habits, you can get return to your original vision by letting your imagination run free, seeing yourself beautiful, lovable, and whole.

Your imagination and desire live at your ideal weight creates a physical desire to take action. Let your imagination go free when you imagine life at your ideal weight. Writing these thoughts down whenever you have them can be powerful reminders in times when your desire is not so clear. Let yourself be creative. You can have so much fun with your own imagination!

Allow yourself to keep exploring your original vision of what it will be like to be thinner. You can build on your original desire by adding new details as you come closer to your ideal weight and more secure in your success. Picture yourself in the kinds of clothes you will be wearing when you reach your ideal weight and plan a new, exciting style for yourself. Think about the colors you will wear and how you'll feel when people begin to notice the changes you've made. Trigger the possibility by using your imagination!

At the time I decided to reduce my weight, tight jeans were very fashionable. I never even considered the possibility that I would ever be able to wear a pair and look the way I wanted to, because I was always too overweight.

It took me several weeks into my own program to allow myself to believe that I could wear a pair of jeans. One day I bought a pair in a size 10, my goal size, and decided to go for it. I'll never forget the day I actually got them up over my hips! It was a sign of progress, but I still couldn't close the zipper. I didn't get discouraged. I kept my intention in mind. After all, I was making progress! I waited for several weeks to try again, and, much to my astonishment, I could zip them up and even button them at the top (if I sucked in my breath). I still couldn't sit down with them on, but I was moving in the right direction. So I took them off, hung them on the closet door, and looked at them every day for three more weeks.

I smile to myself now when I think about how much I wanted to get into those jeans. And then one day it happened. I zipped them up, buttoned the top, sat down…I had done it! I looked at myself in the mirror and gave an excited yell.

I vowed then I would never be overweight again. The feeling of reaching my ideal weight and the pleasure of how I looked to myself was too great to ever go back to anything less than feeling great about my weight and my ability to succeed. I noticed that I felt like I was in control—not only of my weight, but also of my life.

I began to wonder why I had waited so long, and I realized that it was because, up until then, I hadn't believed in myself and my capabilities. By letting go of my extra weight, I came to know a particular state of confidence and inner strength. These feelings tapped the well of my personal power. To this day, I have never gone back to the old habits of eating and eating and eating.

The weight will not come back, because this is not a diet. What you are doing now is not just about reaching your ideal weight. You are discovering how to live the life of inner serenity you have always dreamed about. You are falling in love with the real you. These new awarenesses can help you face your fears in the bright light of spirit.

You are now beginning to align your inner state with your outer action. In the coming weeks you will see change manifest itself spontaneously in your life. Don't try to obsessively control this change. Your job is to take steps day to day that keep your beliefs and desire in line with what you want to manifest in your life.

When you clear away the old habits and open your heart, you create opportunity for new abundance in your life. Allow these gifts to come to you. You don't need to suffer anymore. You deserve to live your potential. You deserve to have your dreams. Believe that, and your life will reflect it back to you like a perfect flower reflected in a bottomless pool of possibility.

Give Gratitude

Remembering to be grateful keeps us aware of how miraculous our existence is. I like to "check in" with different parts of my life from time to time to say "thank you."

Just think, for example, what our bodies do for us every day. Our feet carry us miles and miles.

Oh, thank you feet!

Our breath goes on and on every second and automatically for us every single minute of our lives.

Thank you, breath!

Our heart signals feelings and we cry and feel relief afterward.

Thank you, heart!

We look up to the blue sky and hear birds singing in the trees.

Thank you, eyes! Thank you, ears!

Our bodies are miracles in motion that we often forget to appreciate. We create careers, build houses and raise children, and our bodies stand right beside us every step of the way. Sometimes we only acknowledge our bodies when they don't feel good or when we have an injury. They house our mind and spirit. Without them functioning in perfect harmony we suffer. When they work beautifully, when we care for our bodies and give gratitude for them, we enter a state of oneness, physical and spiritual working together.

One of the most exciting things my seminar students tell me is that as they begin to reach their ideal weight, they become happier people, and that's not just because they are reducing their weight. It's also because they have found a new way of seeing themselves and seeing the world—a new way that casts a light of appreciation and fulfillment on everything they do. Instead of being burdened by life, they can see the blessing of possibility.

Give yourself appreciation for all that you know to be good and true about yourself. Believe that you were created perfect in nature, like a flower that has one path: to grow and bloom. Allow your knowledge and your learning to flow through your body and your mind, like a river that never overflows its banks but gently travels over rocks and reaches its destination in its right time.

Experience every aspect of your life in different and more satisfying ways than when you relied on old habits, resources and messages from the past that are no longer useful in your transformation. Unrestricted by limiting thoughts, attitudes and negative emotions, you can now enjoy a freer and more expansive life.

As you let go of judging others, you can turn inward and each day be renewed with enthusiasm and joy, transforming your heart's desires to that of your own wellbeing and satisfaction. Regardless of the confusion and discord around us all, our trust in a higher power in the universe keeps us serene and peaceful because we believe in a constant source of strength, assurance, and comfort.

You can practice each day, learning and experiencing the rewards of faith. Any number of old habits can delay learning. You can accept yourself just as you are, realizing you always have a positive intention in all that you do. Remember and accept that you are progressing toward being the best of all that, in the best part of your being, you already are.

After you finish this book you will have an understanding of everything you need to walk, step by step, toward your vision, whatever that means for you. That includes a lot more than just reaching your ideal weight. During the seminars I conduct, the final week is always filled with lots of joy and some fear. Nearly every participant loses weight and feels better about the direction of his or her life, and this is cause for celebration. Finishing the seminar, however, is a little scary because now they are challenged with continuing the program on their own, just as you are being challenged now.

Your healthy, spirited body lives in a state of desire that compels you to make decisions and take action toward your own state of wellbeing. We've talked about thought, imagination, decision making, love, the higher self, and many other ideas that give you fulfillment and satisfaction. This learning is something that can only be cultivated through experience and practice.

To align yourself with your intended state of being, begin to align your thoughts with gratitude. If you hold fearlessly to your intended wholeness, your experience will be confirmed as wholeness—being "full-filled" instead of just feeling full. Our bodies don't know the difference between an imagined experience and a real experience.

Our bodies respond to every picture and sound we actually experience, remember experiencing, or imagine experiencing. If before skiing a steep run I construct a picture of flawless skiing, my body believes that I am that skillful, and it responds with excitement and readiness. If I imagine myself going flawlessly through a presentation or an interview, my body and brain respond with more spontaneity and energy. I create a pattern that my mind can follow, and if I believe the pattern and put my full faith in it, my body will respond.

If I wake up every morning and imagine myself at my ideal weight, eating in a way that will support that vision, nurturing my body, paying attention to the messages from my spirit, I've planted a seed that will grow throughout the day.

Seek and You Shall Find

Anyone who is constantly *seeking* will rarely be completely happy. Those who are constantly *finding* tend to be the ones who are fulfilled and find satisfaction in the day to day living. Finding is not something that happens to us. It's an attitude we can consciously choose to cultivate.

The difference between seeking and finding is that seekers always have their eyes on the horizon, but if you ask where they are right now and where they have come since yesterday, they have no idea. They are always focused on their dissatisfaction, where they have to go before they can feel satisfied:

"Yes, I'm happy, but…"

"Of course I'm successful, but…"

"Yes, other people say I have good qualities, but…"

Finders also have their eyes on the horizon. They, too, have visions that they want to reach, but they also know exactly where they are today. They appreciate the journey they are on. They know that they have already come far, and that this—every single day—is a success as large as the moment when they reach that vision on the horizon. Steps along the way create the willingness to go on.

Becoming a finder is something you can choose to do. It is a state of fulfilling your intention toward yourself and your life. It's a way that you can keep yourself enthusiastic about your progress even while you take steps toward your desire. When you're feeling down or you've had a hard day—and we all do—STOP, and ask yourself these questions:

- How can I *find* and have what I am *seeking*?
- How do I want to feel at the end of this day?
- How have I felt my state of excellence before?
- How did I know I was feeling *really* good?

The True Beginning

A key to keeping your ideal weight is being in touch with what you really seek. To do this, you must look carefully at your feelings, study them and learn to relax even with feelings that give rise to feeling over-whelmed. Deep inside yourself, feelings are trying to send a message to the real you, a message about the self you desire to be. To find these feelings, we peel away those layers of judgment and criticism to find the loving, all-accepting self within, the Divine Self.

The Self ignites sparks of feelings. Our experiences and memories ignite sparks of feelings. Our all-knowing, wise hearts send us sparks of feelings. You wake up and see the sun shining and a smile comes to your face. You see a friend and she tells you some good news. You feel a rush of joy. Then the telephone rings and you learn a friend is sick. Your joy gives way to sadness and worry for your friend, thoughts of what you can do to help your friend, hope that she'll be well again soon, and gratitude for your own health. You may feel overwhelmed and fearful about the news. What will the future bring for her? What will the future bring for you? There's no way to know.

So many emotions. These sparks merge in us creating new ideas and new convictions. These sparks can paralyze us. These sparks can also lead us to make new decisions. These sparks can move us toward a path of love and change.

You are a seeker of happiness, peace, and satisfaction. You are just like me. We are the same. We are connected with each other as you read. Sometimes we have only the memories of our connection, but we are still together. As seekers we all lost our way from time to time, or at least we thought we lost our way. We actually came to a fork in the road, or we got confused. We became afraid. Afraid of ourselves, afraid we aren't capable of having our dreams…afraid to try again. We almost gave up, because it seemed easier than going forward. And then…

Something inside ourselves cried for help, yearned for more under-standing. We didn't dare to ask who is that human who cries for help? Who am I really?

Bravo, little bird…now you are ready to feel your wings, to soar from season to season unfolding your wings, developing from a little ball of fluff, soft and fragile, to your freedom to fly. Your freedom to be you.

You have tried everything outside of yourself. You have listened to what others have said was best for you. But it wasn't the best for you, and you realized that the messages from your heart guide you on the path that is your destiny. You, who are the little bird, the seed planted in the universe…planted in love, conceived in love, a living miracle. There are more sides to you than you ever dreamed possible. You are really a multifaceted gem stone. You are not just what you think, not just what you do. You are more than your body, your habits, your role as mother, father, child, and worker. You are a bud ready to blossom. You are ready and willing to learn change and find out who you really are. And you are only love.

Look around you. Look inside you. Listen to your heart.

My creativity flows from within me.
I listen to the Divine message from within, my higher self.
Through learning and a step-by-step process, I reach all that I want.
This day goes well.
Today is a "new shoe day."
Nothing is lost, only transformed.
Every day I am transforming.
I'm riding waves of joy.

About the Author

Mary Bray has for the last 15 years dedicated her life to helping people from around the world reach their perfect weight. Based in Switzerland since the 1980s, her books, programs and private consultations focus on the healing connections in mind, body and spirit.

CPSIA information can be obtained at www.ICGtesting.com
Printed in the USA
LVOW071614100212

268131LV00002B/59/A

9 780595 130382